Urology for Nurses

THEATRE
S.G.H.

Urology for Nurses

J. P. Blandy
MA, DM, MCh, FRCS, FACS
Professor of Urology
London Hospital Medical College,
University of London;
Consultant Urologist
St Peter's Hospitals

J. Moors
SRN, RSCN, SCM
Formerly
Sister
Devonshire Ward
The London Hospital

BLACKWELL SCIENTIFIC PUBLICATIONS

OXFORD LONDON EDINBURGH

BOSTON MELBOURNE

© 1989 by
Blackwell Scientific Publications
Editorial offices:
Osney Mead, Oxford OX2 0EL
 (*Orders*: Tel. 0865-240201)
8 John Street, London WC1N 2ES
23 Ainslie Place, Edinburgh EH3 6AJ
3 Cambridge Center, Suite 208
 Cambridge, Massachusetts 02142, USA
107 Barry Street, Carlton
 Victoria 3053, Australia

First published 1989

Set by Times Graphics, Singapore
Printed and bound in Great Britain
by Butler & Tanner Ltd
Frome and London

DISTRIBUTORS
USA
 The C.V. Mosby Company
 11830 Westline Industrial Drive
 St Louis
 Missouri 63146
 (*Orders*: Tel. 314-872-8370)

Canada
 The C.V. Mosby Company
 5240 Finch Avenue East
 Scarborough, Ontario
 (*Orders*: Tel. 416-298-1588)

Australia
 Blackwell Scientific Publications
 (Australia) Pty Ltd
 107 Barry Street
 Carlton, Victoria 3053
 (*Orders*: Tel. 03-347-0300)

British Library
Cataloguing in Publication Data

Blandy, John P.
 Urology for nurses.
 1. Urological nursing
 I. Title   II. Moors, J.
 616.6'0024613   RC874.7

ISBN 0-632-01686-8

Contents

Preface

The authors have worked together for many years at the London Hospital where urological and nephrological patients are cared for in a single ward area, and where physicians, surgeons and nurses together are responsible for all aspects of urology and nephrology — whether it be torsion, teratoma, transurethral resection or transplantation. During our long association we have both been involved in efforts to raise standards of urological care and in teaching the subject to undergraduate and postgraduate students of both disciplines.

We have long been dissatisfied with existing textbooks for nurses who need a background to their ward experience and a stimulus and pointer to further reading. We have gone to some trouble to use plain English rather than medical jargon, not because we wish to condescend to our readers, but because everyday English is usually more clear, and we are well aware that for some of our readers even English will not be their first language — let alone any of the pretentious jargon which springs from the unhappy union of classical Greek and medieval Latin.

We know all too well that many of our readers will have just come off duty. Their shoes are off. Their tired feet are up on a chair. They have the choice between the television or our textbook; and so we must neither be prosy nor dull. Bristling with its many unsolved problems, urology can be demanding, daunting, and often downright exhausting — but it is certainly never dull; we have tried to communicate our enthusiasm for it.

Many of our readers will be taught in schools which emphasize the 'nursing process', a system for which we have considerable respect. 'Care plans' must, by definition, be individual, but in this book we assume a basic nursing knowledge, and although we attempt to explain any relevant procedures more fully, and refer to coexistent illness when appropriate, our main aim has been to explain the particular problems related to the urological condition and to suggest the role of the nurse in recognizing and coping with these.

J.P.B., J.M.

1 *The urological patient*

Introduction

The patient with a urological disorder

All kinds of patient may have a urological disorder: there are babies with congenital abnormalities; little boys needing circumcision; healthy young men suddenly injured in a motor cycle accident — anxious about the future; mothers with bladders damaged after a difficult birth; women of all ages with incontinence of urine; frail old men distressed with the symptoms of enlargement of the prostate; people with stones, cancer of the kidney, testis and bladder, and those in renal failure who need dialysis or transplantation.

With such a variety the differing needs of patients are endless, and the challenges continual. In urology the nurse is part of a team, much of whose effort is devoted to the prevention of unnecessary renal failure from obstruction or infection that could be relieved. But the work of the team is unique in that if they fail in this, there are the alternatives of dialysis or transplantation.

A nurse needs to know the structure and function of the urinary tract and be able to explain to patients and relatives in language which they can understand what normally happens in their bodies and what has gone wrong.

Patients deserve to know what to expect when they go for a test or an operation: why these procedures are needed, what they are intended to achieve and what they will entail: the more they can participate and understand, the less their anxiety and fear. Equally important for them is to have some idea of how long they are likely to be in hospital, what they should or should not do when they go home, and when they may safely resume their normal activities.

Admission to hospital — general considerations and assessment

Many patients will have been seen several times in their doctor's surgery or the outpatient clinic and by the time they are admitted they will often have undergone several investigations. Some will have had previous in-patient treatment, and will know what to expect, but all will be anxious to

1

know the outcome of any examination or operation, and an understanding attitude to these fears can be reassuring (Fig. 1.1).

Many patients with urological disorders have other serious illnesses: some will have undergone cardiac surgery; some are breathless from emphysema; some have diabetes or disabling arthritis; some are hard of hearing, partially sighted, or confined to a wheelchair. Nurses must use their powers of observation while admitting the patient; they must assess his or her general state and reaction, and make note of any particular difficulties. The most valuable insight comes from listening to the patient and finding out how he or she copes with their disabilities at home. All patients' problems are relevant to their care; all must be considered.

Patients admitted as an emergency are often very ill, in pain, and need urgent treatment for an obstructed bladder or kidney, severe infection or injury. Sometimes the unplanned admission will be for the excited patient summoned to hospital for a long awaited transplant. It is all the more

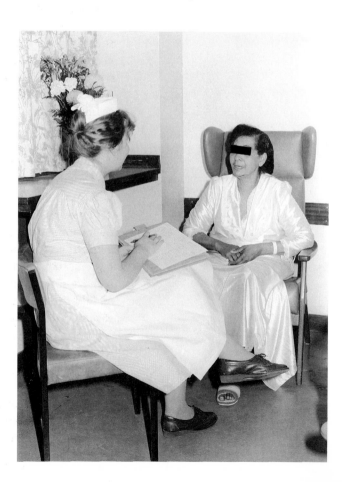

Fig. 1.1 The nurse interviewing a patient on admission.

important that a concise and careful explanation is given to these patients as each procedure is carried out. In an emergency relatives may arrive with the patient or they may need to be notified and called to hospital. They also must be cared for and can often be very helpful in providing information and in comforting the patient. Explaining what is being done will go far to allay their fears.

Admission is also the best time to spot potential difficulties related to discharge, so that plans can be made in plenty of time, e.g. arranging support services at home, booking convalescence, or arranging modifications to the house or flat.

Assessment of the urinary problem

Urological patients have characteristic problems, and nurses need to be familiar with their symptoms — for example, 'I keep wetting myself, I have pain, I keep getting up in the night, I have seen blood in my water, I can't pass my water, I keep on going to the toilet but only pass a little drop each time.'

One needs to find out how long these things have been going on; when and where the pain is experienced; how much bleeding there has been or how bad the incontinence? What has already been done? What does he or she hope will be done now? This must be done discreetly and sensitively, as many patients are extremely embarrassed about these personal matters.

Most important of all — how do these symptoms affect their life? Frequency, pain and incontinence can be socially disabling. Some are prevented from leaving the home or having friends in for a chat. Others dare not pick up small children for fear of incontinence. It may be impossible to go to the theatre, enjoy a pint, travel on a bus, or sit through a business meeting. Many try to restrict their fluid intake to a minimum, however thirsty they may become, to make life bearable. Many become sore from wearing pads.

The plan for care can now be made. Baseline observations will be made of temperature, pulse, respiration, blood pressure, and weight. Urinalysis is performed and an appropriately collected specimen of urine sent to the laboratory for culture and microscopy.

An accurate *fluid chart* will record the *frequency and volume* of urine passed, and its relation to intake. Most patients can record this themselves after a little instruction, passing their urine directly into a measuring container. Make sure that they can read and understand the markings on the container and how to record the chart. This simple input and output chart (Fig. 1.2) will answer two important questions — how

Time	In (ml)	Out (ml)
7.30 a.m.	165	250
8.05		150
8.45		100
11.15	145	
12.00 noon	310	
12.55 p.m.		250
1.15		220
1.50		210
2.30		190
4.00	290	
5.05		100
6.15	1100	
6.30		250
6.45		310
7.30		150
8.05	150	
10.00	150	
11.00	150	
2.00 a.m.		110
2.30		55
3.55		75
5.50		120
	2460	2640

Fig. 1.2 A simple fluid chart can be kept by the patient.

often does he or she empty their bladder, and how much urine is passed each time?

Catheterizing a patient with acute retention may often solve one immediate problem but for patients with frequency who are undergoing investigation or radiotherapy to the bladder, a low bed near the toilet, a bedside commode (Fig. 1.2) or a urinal at hand (Fig. 1.3) may help to provide much needed rest.

An incontinent patient will appreciate the nurse's offer of protection for the bed or suitable pads. A patient with a urostomy may need a supply of appliances or a night drainage bag.

Anyone admitted for 'routine' surgery or investigations should be given an explanation of what these entail and one should try to answer all their questions. When planning the operating list the actual and mental

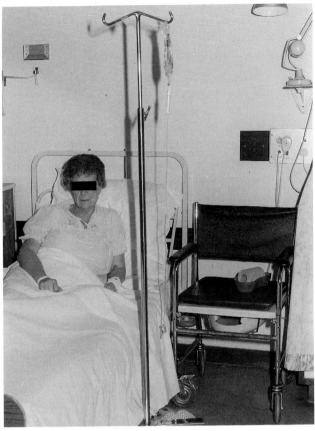

Fig. 1.3 A commode beside the bed may provide rest for the patient with severe frequency.

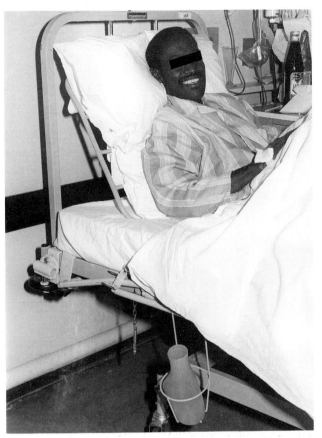

Fig. 1.4 For the man with frequency a urinal may be placed close at hand.

age of the patient should be taken into consideration along with the general medical condition. Unnecessary distress is caused if very young, very old, mentally handicapped or anxious patients are kept waiting without food or drink for a large part of the day before surgery, and this can have adverse effects on their postoperative recovery.

Further reading

Blandy, J. P. (1989) *Lecture Notes on Urology*, 4th edn. Blackwell Scientific Publications, Oxford.

Blandy, J. P. (Ed.) (1976) *Urology*. Blackwell Scientific Publications, Oxford.

Smith, D. R. (Ed.) (1984) *General Urology*, 11th edn. Lange, Los Altos.

Whitfield, H. N. & Hendry, W. F. (1985) *Textbook of Genito-Urinary Surgery*. Churchill Livingstone, Edinburgh.

2 *The kidney — structure and function*

When you hold the living kidney in your hand during a surgical operation it throbs because blood is rushing through it at the rate of half a litre a minute. It is hard to imagine how such a little organ, barely larger than a fist, could have such important work and yet it does one of the most important jobs in the body — maintaining the internal environment.

Ages ago when our remote ancestors crawled out of the sea onto dry land, they preserved inside the waterproof covering of their skin an extracellular fluid surrounding every cell in the body, with the same composition as the ancient sea from which they had emerged. From then onwards, kidneys evolved to make sure that this extracellular fluid preserved exactly the composition of that primeval ocean. The kidneys do this in five ways:

1 They continually *clear the blood of toxic waste* — the most important of which are the by-products of nitrogen metabolism, e.g. urea and creatinine.

2 They adjust the *quantity* of the extracellular fluid by varying the *volume* of urine that is formed.

3 They keep a constant watch on its *quality*, continually adjusting its *acidity* and *salt content* so that the pH and osmolality are kept within very narrow limits of tolerance.

4 They make sure of their own blood supply by adjusting the *blood pressure* with the *renin–angiotensin* mechanism to provide plenty of blood for themselves.

5 They regulate the amount of blood being made by secreting *erythropoietin*, a hormone which stimulates bone marrow to make red cells.

The situation and relations of the kidneys

Each kidney is about 12 cm long. Behind it is the quadratus lumborum muscle, the 12th rib and the lower edge of the pleura (Fig. 2.1). In front are the duodenum and colon — on the right side the second part of the duodenum and the ascending colon; on the left the duodenojejunal flexure and the descending colon. Medial to the kidney are the great vessels; on the right the inferior vena cava, on the left the aorta. The renal artery and vein enter and leave the kidney in front of the renal pelvis (Fig. 2.2).

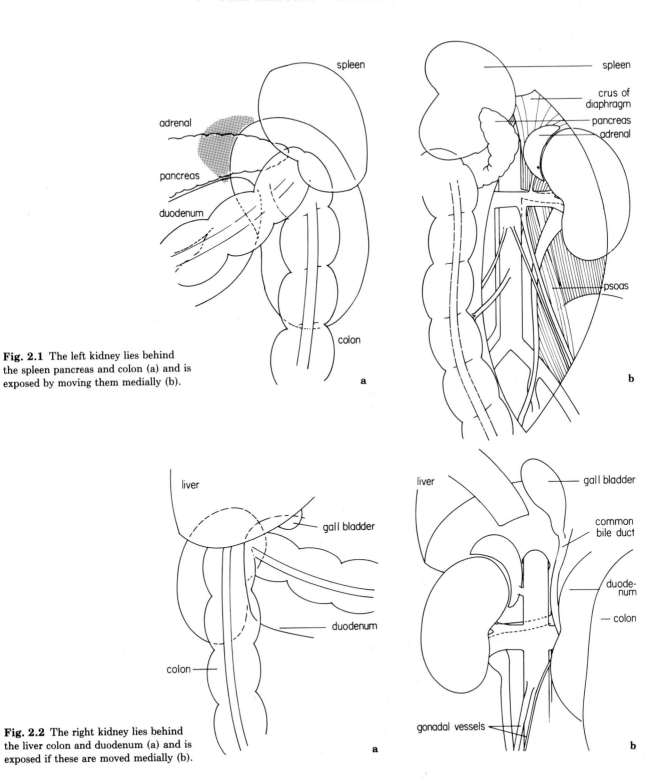

Fig. 2.1 The left kidney lies behind the spleen pancreas and colon (a) and is exposed by moving them medially (b).

Fig. 2.2 The right kidney lies behind the liver colon and duodenum (a) and is exposed if these are moved medially (b).

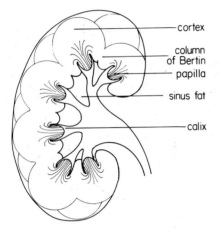

cortex

column of Bertin

papilla

sinus fat

calix

Fig. 2.3 Each kidney is made up of a collection of pyramids each draining into its own papilla.

The basic unit of the kidney — the pyramid

Each kidney is made up of about a dozen *pyramids* (Fig. 2.3). In many mammals, for example, the porpoise, these are clustered like a bunch of grapes and indeed they start like this in the human fetus, but by the time the baby is born the pyramids have been moulded together into the familiar shape of the kidney. However, if you slice an adult kidney open, you can easily make out the pattern of the individual pyramids, each of which is shaped like a bunch of flowers in a vase, with two obvious components — the 'flowers' on the outside or *cortex* (Latin = bark or rind), and the 'stems' on the inside or medulla (Latin = middle) (Fig. 2.4). The cortex and medulla, as opposed to the collecting system of the renal pelvis, are sometimes referred to as the *renal parenchyma* (Greek = infilling or stuffing).

The nephron

To the naked eye the cut surface of the cortex is speckled with little round dots. Under a microscope each dot is seen to be made up of a little coiled up artery the *glomerulus* (Latin = ball of wool). Each glomerulus is surrounded by a hollow bag (*Bowman's capsule*) which empties down a waste-pipe — the *renal tubule* (Fig. 2.5).

As blood flows through the coiled glomerular arteriole, most of its water oozes out into the hollow of Bowman's capsule, carrying with it the things that normally dissolve in water, e.g. glucose, salt, and urea — the *solutes*. The blood cells and protein molecules are filtered off by the

Fig. 2.4 The pyramid has the structure of a bunch of flowers (glomeruli) whose stems (collecting tubules) are stuck into a vase (calix).

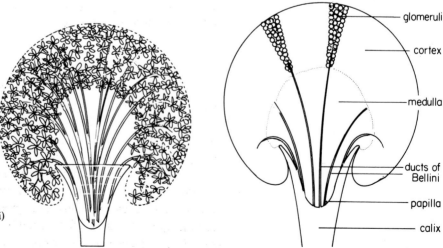

glomeruli

cortex

medulla

ducts of Bellini

papilla

calix

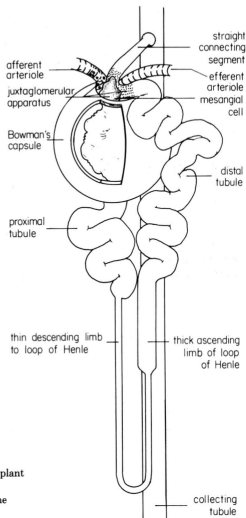

Fig. 2.5 The nephron is the basic renal unit: it comprises the filtering plant of the glomerulus inside Bowman's capsule, and the processing plant (the tubule).

basement membrane (Fig. 2.6) which only allows water and solutes — the *glomerular filtrate* — to pour down the waste pipe of the renal tubule.

Each tubule (Fig. 2.7) is made of two twisted parts (*the proximal and distal convoluted tubule*) separated by a long narrow part bent like a hairpin — the *loop of Henle*. The longer of these hairpin loops dangle down among the collecting tubules in the medulla.

The glomerulus and its tubule work together as a unit — the *nephron*. The tubules draw back just enough water from the filtrate to keep the osmolality of the extracellular fluid in the body always the same, and just enough of each solute that the body requires; they let go all the rest. The

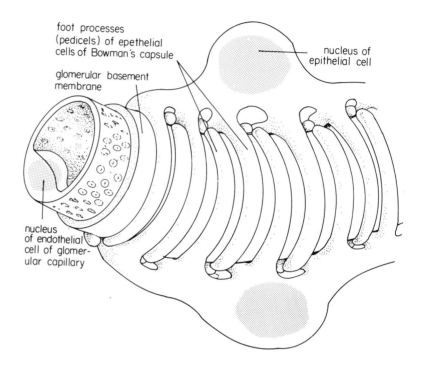

foot processes
(pedicels) of epethelial
cells of Bowman's capsule

nucleus of
epithelial cell

glomerular basement
membrane

nucleus
of endothelial
cell of glomer-
ular capillary

Fig. 2.6 The basement membrane is a
filter lying between the sieve-like cells of
the glomerular capillary and the
supporting struts of the lining cells of
Bowman's capsule.

control of the amount of water reabsorbed is governed by the anterior
pituitary gland which secretes an antidiuretic hormone according to the
osmolality of the blood that reaches it. The tubules also adjust the acidity
of the extracellular fluid by varying the amount of hydrogen ions that they
actively pump out. All the soluble waste materials, especially urea, are
allowed to escape in the urine.

The two different parts of the kidney that are so obvious when it is
sliced across — the cortex and medulla — remind one of its two different
functions: filtration in the cortex and processing the filtrate in the
medulla. These two parts of the kidney may be affected differently in
different diseases. In nephritis the glomeruli are inflamed and damaged so
that filtration is restricted or ineffective. In prolonged *obstruction* the
medulla may be destroyed but the cortex continues to make glomerular filtrate which is not then properly processed, and as a result a
large volume of dilute urine is passed and valuable salt lost from the
body.

The collecting system

The renal tubules enter collecting ducts, about a dozen in each pyramid —
i.e. a dozen flowers in the bunch. Each duct opens on the tip of the renal

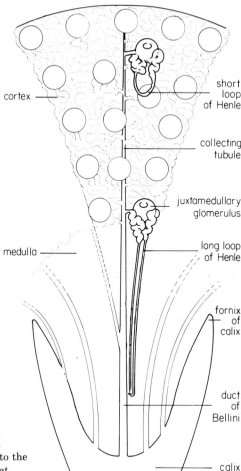

cortex

short
loop
of Henle

collecting
tubule

juxtamedullary
glomerulus

medulla

long loop
of Henle

fornix
of
calix

duct
of
Bellini

calix

Fig. 2.7 The nephrons are arranged like corn on the cob — those nearer to the medulla having long hairpin loops that dangle down into the renal papilla.

papilla (Latin = nipple). The papilla protrudes into a cavity shaped like a wineglass — the *calix* (Greek = chalice or wine-cup). There is one calix for each papilla and pyramid. The complete set of a dozen calices enters a common basin — the *renal pelvis* (Latin = basin) which empties down its waste-pipe — the *ureter* — down which the urine is pumped into the *bladder* (Fig. 2.8).

Calices, pelvis, ureter and bladder are made of smooth muscle lined with waterproof *urothelium*. Their muscular wall pumps the urine from the kidney down to the bladder by rhythmical peristaltic contractions whose tempo is governed by pacemakers in the calices: peristalsis is faster when there is more urine to be pumped out of the kidney.

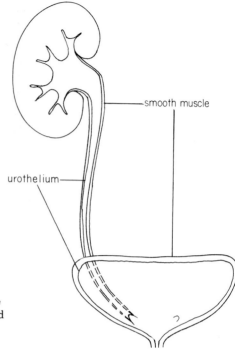

Fig. 2.8 The collecting system of the kidney — the calices, pelvis ureter and bladder — are made of a continuous muscular wall lined by urothelium.

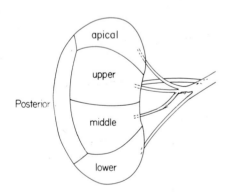

Fig. 2.9 Each renal artery has five branches, each supplying one segment of the kidney.

Blood supply

Arteries

Each renal artery comes straight off the aorta and divides into five branches, one for each main segment of the kidney (Fig. 2.9). Each segmental artery subdivides again and again until the cortex is reached where the arterioles form the 'balls of wool' in the glomeruli. After much of its water and solutes have been filtered out, the blood is passed on into the capillary bed around the collecting tubules where just enough of the water and solutes for the needs of the body are recovered. When the blood finally reaches the renal vein it has been cleansed of all its waste products, and its pH and osmolality have been adjusted exactly to the requirements of the body.

Regulation of blood pressure

Just where the renal arteriole begins to coil up to form the glomerulus a little group of special cells are placed (the *juxtaglomerular cells*, Fig. 2.5). These constantly monitor the blood pressure. If the blood pressure falls, they secrete *renin*, an enzyme which converts *angiotensinogen* — an inactive plasma protein — into *angiotensin I* (Fig. 2. 10). This is carried off in the renal vein, round the heart, to the lungs where another enzyme turns it into *angiotensin II.* Angiotensin II is taken back to the heart, and on to the adrenal gland, where it stimulates the adrenal cortex to secrete *aldosterone.* This raises the blood pressure by narrowing the peripheral blood vessels so as to increase their resistance and causing the renal tubules to retain more salt and water in order to expand the blood volume.

The renal arteries are 'end arteries'

None of the five segmental branches of the renal artery join up with each other as in most organs of the body so if one of them is blocked, the entire segment of the kidney will die (Fig. 2.11). This may happen if a clot from a mitral valve is swept off in the bloodstream and gets stuffed tightly into a renal artery; the resulting dead segment is called an *infarct* (Latin,

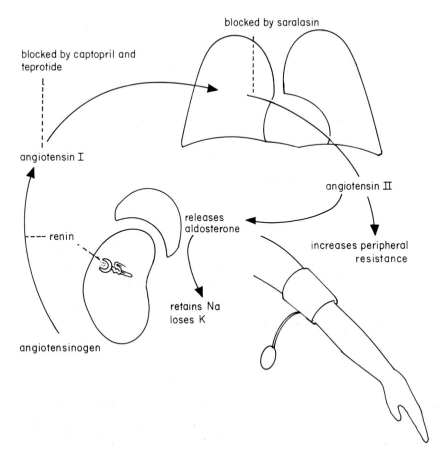

Fig. 2.10 With a fall in blood pressure the juxtaglomerular cells release renin which sets off a chain of events that end up by raising the blood pressure again.

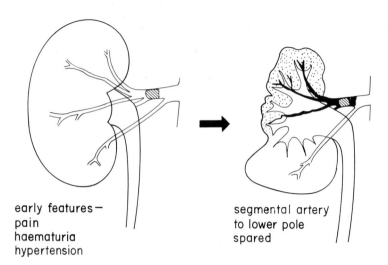

early features—
pain
haematuria
hypertension

segmental artery
to lower pole
spared

Fig. 2.11 Infarction of all but the lower segment of the kidney.

infarcere = to stuff). This can be made use of deliberately in the treatment of renal injury, when a plug of fibrin is sometimes injected into a segmental artery to stop haemorrhage.

Veins

The renal veins are very big. They have no valves where they join the vena cava, so accidental haemorrhage from the renal vein at operation can be fearsome.

Lymphatics

In addition to veins, the kidneys have a profuse system of lymphatics through which urine may escape into the circulation if the ureter is obstructed, acting as a useful safety-valve. Less safe, unfortunately, bacteria may enter the circulation by this route when there is both obstruction and infection.

Nerves

Many fine nerves go to and from the kidneys but even today nobody knows what they do; possibly they transmit pain, and when nothing else seems to stop a kidney hurting, an attempt may be made to provide relief by cutting them — but such relief seldom lasts long. All these nerves are necessarily severed at transplantation, and yet the kidney works perfectly well; evidently they have nothing to do with peristalsis of the calices, pelvis and ureter.

Further reading

Blandy, J. P. (1989) *Lecture Notes on Urology*, 4th edn. Blackwell Scientific Publications, Oxford.

Graves, F. T. (1971) *The Arterial Anatomy of the Kidney.* Wright, Bristol.

Tanagho, E. (1984) Anatomy of the genitourinary tract. In *General Urology*, 11th edn, ed. Smith, D. R., pp. 1–13. Lange, Los Altos, California.

3 The kidney — investigations

Clinical examination

The kidney is so well tucked away that it is only when it is very large or the patient very thin that it can be felt by abdominal palpation and in practice urology has to rely on other methods for making a diagnosis.

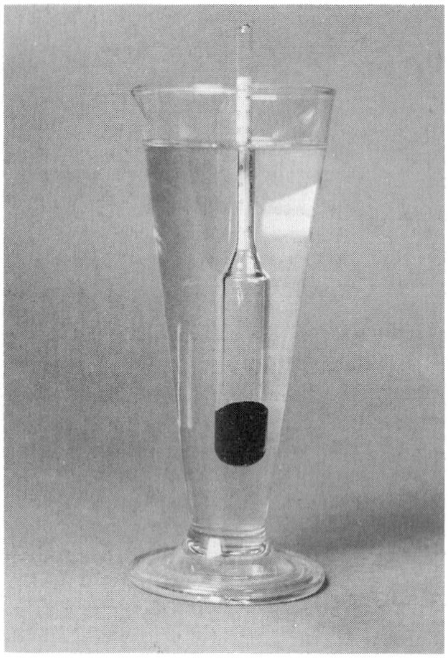

Testing the urine

Specific gravity

A specimen of urine is collected into a clean glass container, in which a hydrometer is allowed to float, and the specific gravity is read off from the markings on its stem (Fig. 3.1). The specific gravity of the urine varies with the number of ions dissolved in it. When the patient is dehydrated, concentrated urine with a high specific gravity (up to 1040) is formed; when the patient is overhydrated the dilute urine may have a specific gravity as low as 1003. When the renal tubules are damaged and unable to process the glomerular filtrate, the urine has an unvarying fixed specific gravity of about 1010.

'Stix' paper strips are now available for estimating the specific gravity. A chemical effect — the relation between the pKa change of polyelectrolytes and ionic concentration — causes an indicator to change colour. This is sufficiently accurate for most purposes and has the advantage of needing only a small quantity of urine.

Fig. 3.1 A hydrometer used to measure the specific gravity of urine.

pH

The strip of paper is impregnated with the dyes methyl red and bromthymol blue, which change colour according to the pH of the urine and are accurate to 0.5 pH unit in the range pH 5 to pH 8.5. Infection with microorganisms which turn urea into ammonia, for example, *Proteus mirabilis*, produces a very alkaline urine. Patients who always make a very acid urine are prone to form uric acid calculi. When the renal medulla is damaged the urine remains persistently neutral, about pH 7.

16

Glucose

The test paper contains the two enzymes glucose oxidase and peroxidase, and the chemical potassium iodide. The glucose oxidase liberates hydrogen peroxide from glucose, and the peroxidase causes it to react with the potassium iodide to produce a brown colour. If glucose is discovered, a 'clinitest' may be performed to measure its quantity.

Protein

The paper is impregnated with tetrabromphenol blue, which goes green in the presence of protein. Because it relies on the change in colour of an indicator it is not reliable when the urine is very acid or very alkaline.

Two older methods can be used:

1 Boil the urine: if a cloud forms, add a drop of acetic acid. If the cloud remains it is due to protein.

2 Add a drop of 25% salicylsulphonic acid to the urine: a white cloud forms if protein is present.

Sometimes it is important to know if there has been a leak of protein through the glomerular basement membrane. The urine is collected over a 24-hour period and its protein accurately measured in the laboratory; anything more than 50 mg of protein per 24 hours is abnormal.

Blood

The paper contains two ingredients: cumene peroxidase and tetramethylbenzidine. Haemoglobin catalyses a reaction between them to produce a range of colour from orange to dark green. The test detects free haemoglobin, so a positive finding calls for microscopical examination of the urine to see if red cells are present. It is a sensitive test and can detect as few as five red cells per ml — which is only twice the amount that may be found in normal urine. If the container into which the urine has been passed is contaminated with hypochlorite or povidone iodine sterilizing solutions there may be a false positive result. Any haematuria must be investigated further.

Urine culture

Many patients will be undergoing surgery, investigations that require catheterization, or other invasive procedures which may either stir up an unsuspected pre-existing infection of the urinary tract, or introduce new organisms. Clinical symptoms of urinary infection may develop with alarming speed, and it is helpful to be forewarned, and to know what organisms if any, are present in the urine on admission. A catheter or mid-stream specimen of urine should be sent to the laboratory at the earliest opportunity from every patient on admission.

Urine is an excellent culture medium and easily contaminated by dust from the ward or by the skin. At room temperature these contaminants grow rapidly, so any specimen of urine must either be cultured at once or put into a refrigerator until it can be sent to the laboratory to prevent the contaminants from multiplying.

Methods of collection of urine specimens

Mid-stream urine — MSU

The collection of a mid-stream urine specimen is often more easily said than done especially if the patient is obese, a baby, someone unable to understand instructions, incontinent, or confined to bed. Quite often a 'clean-catch' specimen is the best that can be achieved, and the specimen should be labelled accordingly.

The *male patient* is instructed to wash and dry his hands, retract the foreskin, and clean the meatus with swabs and clean water. After passing some urine into the toilet or a jug, he directs the mid-stream into a sterile container and then continues to empty his bladder into the toilet. He replaces the lid on the container without touching the inside.

The *female patient* holds her labia apart with one hand, and cleans the meatus with swabs by wiping from front to back. She may find it easier to catch the mid-stream urine into a sterile receiver or jug, and later transfer it carefully into the specimen pot. If the patient is using a bedpan a sterile receptacle may be put into the pan for a 'clean-catch' specimen.

A *baby* poses more difficulties: vigilance on the part of the mother or nurse is necessary to catch a mid-stream specimen, but there are certain useful tricks. Tapping lightly on the suprapubic region may initiate micturition, as may the shock of sitting on a cold surface — so that it is a good idea to have a container handy when the baby is being weighed. Small, sterile bags are available for collecting urine from babies. After washing the perineal area and drying it carefully, the adhesive bag is stuck round the meatus and the specimen is transferred to the sterile container as soon as possible after it has been passed.

If a urine specimen is needed urgently from a sick baby or a toddler suspected of having a urinary infection, it may be safely obtained by the doctor by *suprapubic aspiration* of the distended bladder. With the baby lying on its back, the suprapubic area is cleaned with antiseptic and a very fine needle attached to a syringe is introduced at right angles to the skin in the midline.

Catheter urine specimens

At the time of catheterization, urine is collected directly into the specimen container. Catheters are not passed merely to collect a specimen. When there is an indwelling catheter, the specimen is aspirated via the 'sampling port' — a sleeve of rubber on the drainage tubing which seals the puncture site — after cleaning it with an alcohol-impregnated swab. The tube is held in a loop so that urine collects in this section, and a needle and syringe are used to aspirate the specimen (Fig. 3.2).

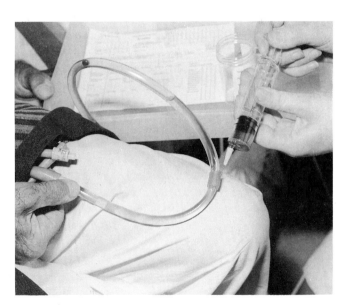

Fig. 3.2 Urine is aspirated through the self-sealing rubber sleeve on the urine drainage tubing.

When there is no sampling port in a latex catheter it may be clamped momentarily, and the catheter itself cleaned and punctured — taking care to avoid the balloon channel.

Catheters must never be left clamped off without specific instructions: it is all too easy to be called away and forget to return, and in the meantime obstruction to the free flow of urine gives rise to back-pressure which easily leads to septicaemia. Because it is so easy to allow airborne organisms to enter the culture medium of the urine inside the catheter, catheters should only be disconnected when there is some special reason — and never merely to obtain a specimen of urine.

Specimens from urinary stomas

A specimen from a stoma is obtained by removing the appliance and gently cleaning the stoma with clean water or saline. Usually the spurt of urine can be caught in a sterile specimen container but sometimes it is necessary to pass a small Jaques catheter into the stoma for about 5 cm and aspirate the urine with a syringe.

Culturing the urine

Commercially available slides coated with culture media may be dipped into the urine, drained off, and placed in an incubator. After 24 hours a glance at the slide will show whether or not there is a significant growth of organisms (Fig. 3.3).

In hospital practice most urine samples will be sent to the central laboratory where the microorganisms are counted, identified, and their antibiotic sensitivity determined. It is always necessary to get the specimen to the laboratory as soon as possible otherwise contaminant microorganisms will multiply at room temperature, and give a misleading result. When there is unavoidable delay, the urine must be put in the refrigerator to prevent this. (Put it in the compartment for medicines — not the ice-tray.)

Urine cytology

Urine formed in the middle of the day — not the urine that has remained in the bladder overnight — is collected into a container to which an equal

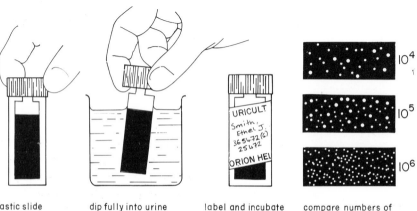

Fig. 3.3 Use of the dip slide method for culturing urine.

plastic slide coated with culture medium

dip fully into urine

label and incubate for 16–24 hours at about 3°C

compare numbers of colonies with standard chart

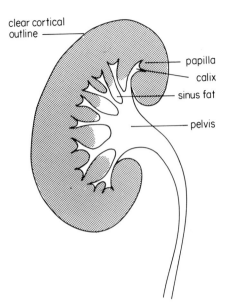

Fig. 3.4 When an X-ray is taken as soon as the contrast medium reaches the renal tubules an image of the cortex is obtained — the nephrogram.

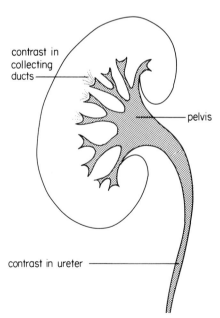

Fig. 3.5 Ten minutes or so later the contrast outlines the calices pelvis and ureter — the urogram.

volume of 10% formalin is added to preserve the cells in the urine. The specimen is centrifuged in the laboratory and the deposit is smeared on a slide and stained to show malignant cells.

X-rays

X-rays might injure a fetus, so except in an emergency, women of child-bearing age are only X-rayed in the first 10 days after the last menstrual period.

A plain abdominal X-ray (kidneys-ureters-bladder or KUB film) will show hazy soft tissue shadows of the kidneys and bladder, but are useful in detecting calcium-containing stones. To show up the urinary tract a radio-opaque contrast medium is used.

The intravenous urogram (IVU)

Intravenous urography is indicated in the investigation of haematuria, stone disease, possible obstruction, and to localize the kidneys before a renal biopsy. It is therefore one of the most common of all urological investigations and its underlying principles are important.

Iodine is opaque to X-rays, but very toxic. If it is made safe by being bound to benzoic acid, the resulting *iodobenzoate* contrast medium can be given intravenously in large doses. As soon as it reaches the kidney it begins to filter out of the glomeruli into the proximal tubules and gives a clear picture of the cortex of the kidney — the *'nephrogram'* (Fig. 3.4).

A few minutes later the filtered iodobenzoate is being concentrated in the tubules and fills the collecting system (Fig. 3.5) so that within 15 minutes one has a complete picture of the urinary tract from calices to bladder; this is the *'intravenous urogram'* — the basic investigation in urology.

Preparations for an IVU

DEHYDRATION

The density of the X-ray shadow in the IVU depends on the concentration of the iodobenzoate in the tubules. The more water reabsorbed from the glomerular filtrate, the clearer will be the X-ray picture, and dehydration may give a slight improvement. It has become routine to forbid fluids for 6 hours before an IVU. In general, this is marginally useful, but at times it can be both silly and dangerous. It can be silly when one needs an answer urgently — the same increase in density of the X-ray shadow may be obtained merely by giving more of the iodobenzoate intravenously. It can be dangerous for uraemic patients who may already be dehydrated and unable to concentrate their urine because of diabetes or tubular damage, and when IVUs have to be done repeatedly, since excessive doses of iodobenzoate may damage the tubules. Dehydration is forbidden in myeloma where overconcentrating the glomerular filtrate may clog up the tubules.

Because gas in the bowel may obscure the shadow of the contrast medium in the collecting system, a purgative is often given to empty the intestine. This can be equally silly and dangerous. It is silly in the normal person who has had his bowels open and is up and about; he is unlikely to be full of wind. It can be dangerous in a patient who gets severe side-effects from purgatives and in ureteric colic when the bowel is always distended with gas. Many a much needed IVU has been thoughtlessly refused on the grounds that 'the patient is not properly prepared'.

Many patients are apprehensive about undergoing an IVU and it will help them greatly if you take a little time to explain what the investigation entails and what it hopes to show. Parental consent is necessary before an IVU is done in children.

Sometimes, to fill out the calices, the ureters are compressed by tightening a broad band on the abdomen for a few minutes — which some patients find uncomfortable.

Dangers of intravenous urography

IVU is useful and often ordered so one must be aware of its dangers.

LOCAL IRRITATION

The iodobenzoate contrast medium is so concentrated that it inevitably irritates the vein, usually causing no more than a little discomfort at the site of injection, but sometimes this irritation causes pain right up the arm and into the shoulder. Occasionally the chemical irritation may be so severe as to cause thrombosis of the vein and the day after the injection the patient notices a red, tender cord along the line of the vein which persists for 10 to 14 days. Patients are often worried by this aseptic chemical thrombosis, and fear that it signifies infection. A careful explanation and an appropriate analgesic is far better than wasting time with poultices which are as useless as they are messy.

This same irritative effect of the contrast medium is noticed at once if it is injected outside the vein by mistake. There is a very painful inflammation at the site of the injection not due to infection, but to chemical irritation. It usually resolves within a few days but occasionally is followed by ulceration of the skin and so it must be documented at the time.

SYSTEMIC EFFECTS

When intravenous contrast medium is given rapidly most patients feel sick and hot. Some have a transient headache and a few may vomit. This innocent if unpleasant pharmacological reaction should not be confused with *allergy*, which is potentially very dangerous.

Allergic reactions vary in degree. Most of them are *minor* — some swelling of the lips, a mild urticarial rash, or a minor asthmatic attack — all quickly relieved by the antihistamine chlorpheniramine maleate (Piriton). The important thing is to note that an allergic reaction has occurred, and warn the patient, for the next time the reaction may be by no means minor.

Major reactions are of two kinds, which may occur singly or together. In the first, there is sudden onset of *oedema* which affects the lips, face and throat so rapidly that the patient may choke to death within seconds. The prompt passage of an endotracheal tube may save life, but there may be nobody there with the right skill and experience to do this. In the last resort, rather than allow the patient to suffocate as large a needle as possible should be thrust through the cricothyroid membrane (Fig. 3.6). It may let in enough air to save life, and give time for expert help to arrive.

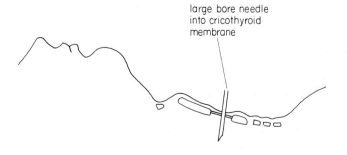

large bore needle into cricothyroid membrane

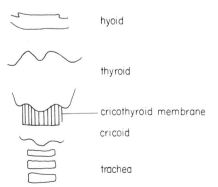

hyoid

thyroid

cricothyroid membrane

cricoid

trachea

Fig. 3.6 In suffocation from acute laryngeal oedema a large needle passed through the cricothyroid membrane to let in air may be life-saving.

The second kind of allergic response is sudden *vasodilatation* leading to a catastrophic fall in blood pressure, unconsciousness, cessation of respiration, and cardiac arrest. First, slip in an airway (Fig. 3.7) and get air into the lungs by mouth to mouth respiration, preferably using an Ambu bag and oxygen. If the pulse cannot be felt, have a colleague start external cardiac massage. 1 ml of 0.1% adrenaline and 100 mg hydrocortisone should be given intravenously the moment the first warning of collapse is seen. The resuscitation team should be summoned who will take an ECG to detect ventricular fibrillation, for which external difibrillation may be needed.

Millions of IVUs are done every year and in every million four will be fatal. Wherever IVUs are done, certain precautions must be followed:

1 Even a minor allergic symptom after iodobenzoate contrast medium rules out a second injection. Note that it is no good testing for 'iodine sensitivity' with skin tests; the allergen is the entire iodobenzoate molecule, not the free iodine. Today there are newer contrast media which are believed to be less likely to provoke an attack, but even these should be used with every precaution at hand.

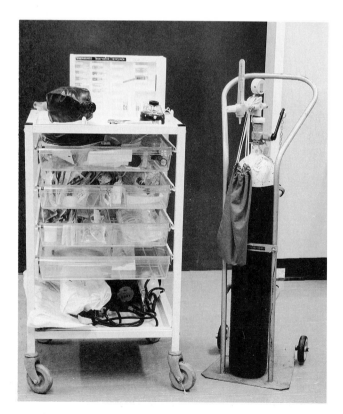

Fig. 3.7 Equipment for resuscitation: 0.1% adrenaline, hydrocortisone, an airway, an Ambu bag and a full cylinder of oxygen.

2 Wherever contrast medium is to be injected, make sure that the minimum equipment for resuscitation is at hand, i.e. 0.1% adrenaline, hydrocortisone, an airway, an Ambu bag and a full oxygen cylinder. Check where it is kept, and how the resuscitation team can be summoned.

Tomography

The film and the X-ray tube are mounted on a beam that swings above and below the kidney on an axle which is level with the kidney (Fig. 3.8). The exposure is made as the beam swings, so that only the kidney remains steady while the other tissues disappear in a gray blur. This gives a picture of a slice through the kidney (Greek, *tomo* = cut) (Fig. 3.9).

Computer assisted tomography — CT scanning

This also gives pictures of slices of the body, but the image is built up in a different way which outlines soft tissues that are not shown in conventional X-rays.

In an ordinary X-ray, electrons are shot through the patient onto a screen which glows like a TV screen with visible light when electrons strike it, and the light is recorded on photographic film. The light and dark shadows in the X-ray depend on how difficult it is for the electrons to pass through the different tissues of the body. This traditional combination of electron, fluorescent screen and photograph is a relatively

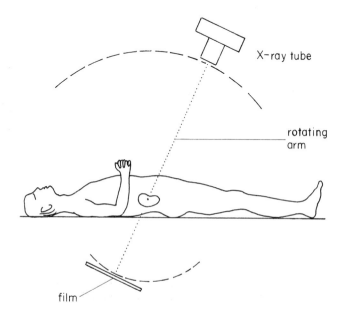

Fig. 3.8 The X-ray tube and the film swing on an axle so that only the tissues on the level of the axle remain in focus — the rest are blurred — giving a slice through the kidney.

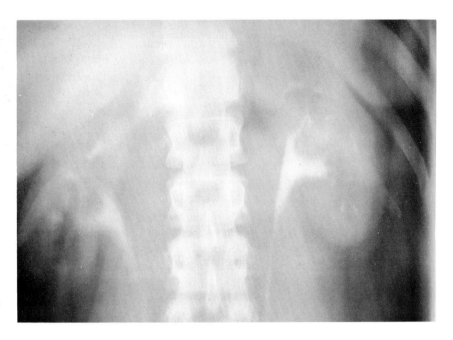

Fig. 3.9 A typical tomogram which shows the soft tissue outline of the kidney and blurs the surrounding tissues.

primitive way of detecting small differences in the beam of electrons and today much more sensitive electronic devices are available. These are placed in a ring around the patient, while the tube is rotated, shining the beam of electrons onto one detector after another. The succession of signals are then analyzed by a computer which presents the information as a series of slices through the patient. Very slight differences in density between one soft tissue and another are clearly defined, giving clear pictures of organs that are indistinguishable by conventional X-rays (Fig. 3.10).

Preparation for CT scan

Patients need to be warned that they must take fluids only for 6 hours prior to the CT scan. Sometimes even better pictures are obtained by using contrast media in the bowel and urinary tract, so they may be asked to drink a litte gastrografin in water about one and a half hours before the investigation to define the bowel more clearly, and an intravenous injection as in an IVU may be given to enhance the shadows of the kidneys, ureters and bladder. The test itself is quite painless but it can be uncomfortable for the patient to lie still on the couch during the test — and some feel a little claustrophobic from the machine that surrounds them.

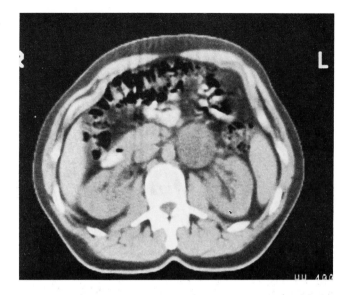

Fig. 3.10 Computerized tomogram showing outlines of soft tissues which would be indistinguishable in an ordinary radiograph.

Angiography

If the whole dose of contrast medium is injected directly into the renal artery it shows all its branches, big and small. In some disorders such as polycystic disease or renal cell carcinoma the change in the normal pattern may be characteristic (Fig. 3.11). Angiography is necessary before live kidney donation to demonstrate the anatomy of the potential donor arterial system, and is often used in the diagnosis of swellings in the region of the kidney.

Preparation and care

Patients need a careful explanation of the procedure and will need to give their informed consent. They will usually need some preliminary sedation.

Both groins must be shaved. In the usual technique of angiography, a thin flexible guidewire is inserted through a needle in the femoral artery, and over the guidewire a thin tube is passed and manoeuvred up the aorta and into the renal artery under X-ray control, and contrast medium injected very rapidly. There is usually a momentary unpleasant sensation of warmth and nausea, and the noise of the mechanism which changes the X-ray plates can be rather startling. Afterwards there may be a bruise in the groin.

After an angiogram the patient must rest in bed for 24 hours. For the first 6 to 8 hours the site of puncture is checked every 30 minutes for

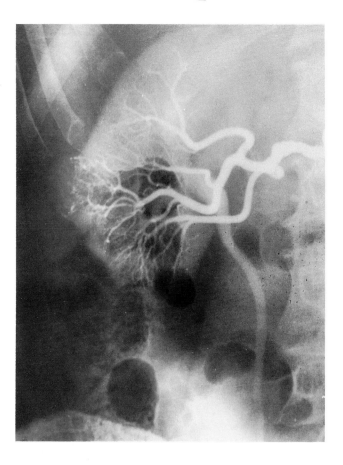

Fig. 3.11 A renal angiogram showing a small cancer on its lateral border.

bleeding and haematoma formation, together with pulse, blood pressure and the pedal pulses on the side of the puncture since the femoral artery is sometimes damaged by the guidewire.

The image of the arteries can be improved by photographing a negative of the preliminary plain film against the positive of the angiogram. This subtracts the images of the bones and gas shadows that may otherwise confuse the picture of the blood vessels and is called *subtraction angiography* (Fig. 3.12).

Digital vascular imaging

Today a computer can do the same trick of subtracting the background and at the same time exaggerate the density of the image, giving a reasonable angiogram without the need to pass a catheter into the renal artery — or at least a much finer one.

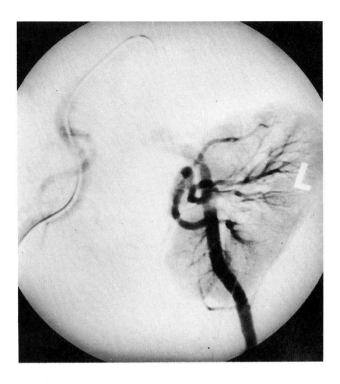

Fig. 3.12 Subtraction angiogram: this shows the blood vessels of a renal transplant which would otherwise be difficult to see against the shadow of the bony pelvis.

Ultrasound

Sound waves — as any porpoise knows — travel very well through water. Bounced off submarines, shoals of fish, and the sea floor, they are used in marine sonar all over the world. Sound waves of ultra high frequency (*ultrasound*) which are inaudible to the human ear, are used to scan the inside of the body. Ultrasound has the advantage that it uses no ionizing radiation, causes no pain, and requires no potentially allergic contrast media. It is especially useful in showing whether a space-occupying renal mass is solid as in cancer or fluid-containing as in a cyst (Fig. 3.13). The patient has to lie still while the ultrasound probe is passed over and over the area to be scanned. The jelly used to obtain good contact between the probe and the skin is easily removed afterwards with a towel.

When scanning the pelvis with ultrasound it helps to have the bladder filled with urine, so the patient may be asked to drink extra fluid and refrain from passing water — which is such a natural instinct when one goes off to another place. An indwelling catheter may have to be clamped off — but remembering the risk of back pressure and septicaemia one must first check with the medical staff that this is safe.

Using a thin ultrasonic probe inserted in the rectum clear pictures may

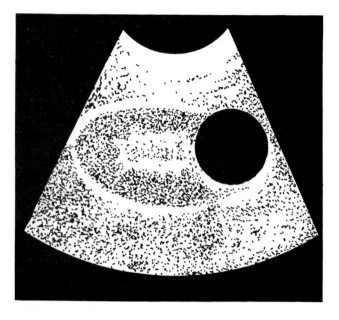

Fig. 3.13 Ultrasound showing an echo-free renal cyst.

be obtained of the prostate. This procedure, which is mildly unpleasant, will be explained very carefully to the patient ahead of time.

Nuclear magnetic resonance (NMR)

Pictures which at first glance resemble those from the CT scanner can be obtained by a new technique which does not use X-rays. Instead the picture is built up by a method which detects the energy given off by the spinning atoms of the tissues of the body after they have been subjected to a very intense magnetic field which is then switched off. The pictures that are provided by NMR distinguish different types of tissue, and even between areas of disease (such as cancer or infarction) within an organ (Fig. 3.14). At the time of writing there are relatively few of these NMR imaging instruments in hospitals, but there is little doubt that within a few years it will become a standard method, particularly in the evaluation of the response of cancer to chemotherapy.

The functions of the kidney

Glomerular filtration

Today we use the expression 'renal function tests' rather loosely. Most of them only measure the glomerular filtration rate (GFR). Some solutes are

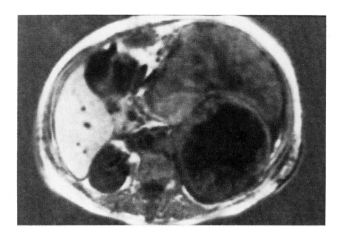

Fig. 3.14 Nuclear magnetic resonance tomogram (courtesy of Dr G. Bidder).

completely cleared from the blood in one passage through the kidney. One of them — creatinine — is easy to measure in blood and urine, and so one may calculate how much blood has been *cleared* per minute and so the glomerular filtration rate (GFR) is usually expressed as the clearance of creatinine in ml per min.

While it is easy enough to measure the concentrations of creatinine in the blood and the urine, a small error in collecting the urine over 24 hours will mean a big error in the result, and in a busy hospital ward it is difficult to be sure that every drop of urine has been collected over a 24-hour period. Only if the urine collection is accurate is the test of any value.

Explain to the patient why the bladder must be empty at the beginning and the end of the collection and why every drop of urine must be saved. Accurate timing of the collection is important since the result is expressed in ml/min. An accurately timed 20- or 21-hour collection is better than an inaccurately timed 24-hour collection. An easy method is to note the time and mark it on the bottle at the start of the collection when the bladder is emptied and the urine discarded. The last specimen is put in the container at exactly the same time the next day.

When the patient is in bed and has a catheter, ask him or her to remind the nurse who takes away the bed-pan or urine that a 24-hour collection is in progress, and write a message on the bag and the fluid chart as additional reminders.

The same answer may be given by injecting a radioactive isotope that is known to be cleared entirely by glomerular filtration, and measuring how quickly it disappears from the blood. A suitable substance is radioactive chromium (^{51}Cr) attached to a short chain of amino acids (ethylenediaminotetra-acetic acid — EDTA). It is given intravenously, and the rate at which the radioactivity disappears is measured either by taking two samples of blood at accurately timed intervals 75 minutes apart, or by placing a Geiger counter over the forearm. Either method avoids the errors that arise from incomplete collection of urine.

Measuring renal tubular function

Two of the functions of the tubule can be measured: (1) its ability to acidify the urine, and (2) to concentrate it.

The acid load test

Explain the test carefully to the patient. Two 1-hour specimens of urine over a period of 2 hours are first collected. Then the patient is given a large loading dose of ammonium chloride, 100 g/kg body (in gelatin-coated capsules — because it is so disgusting) along with a litre of water in one hour. (It often makes them vomit, in which case the test is invalidated). After 3 hours, a third 1-hour collection of urine is made. Renal tubules that are working properly will promptly get rid of the surplus hydrogen ions and the pH of the urine will fall below pH 5.3, with a titratable acidity >25 mEq/min of ammonium. As with creatinine clearance the timings must be very carefully recorded to avoid errors. In practice the test is so unpleasant that it is seldom used.

The urine concentration test

This tests the capacity of the tubule to concentrate urine either in response to 6 hours without water or a dose of pitressin tannate (5 units s.c.) which contains the *antidiuretic hormone* (see p. 10). The specific gravity of the urine is measured in each specimen over the next 3 hours and should reach 1032 if the tubules are working properly. The urine concentration test is also so unpleasant that it is hardly ever used in practice; it is futile in patients already in renal failure and dangerous in those with multiple myeloma.

DMSA imaging

In practice, because the previous two methods of evaluating renal tubular function are so unsatisfactory, when it is necessary to know about the function of the tubules a renogram is performed using 99m Tc dimercaptosuccinic acid (DMSA) which is secreted by the renal tubules so that its uptake measures the total quantity of functioning tubular tissue.

Tests of the function of the collecting system

When we want to know if urine is being obstructed in its passage out of the renal pelvis and down the ureter it is usual to rely on the image provided by the IVU, but there are times when this can be deceiving; a dilated pelvis and ureter may be baggy because they were just made that way, or have become tired and floppy through disease.

The usual iodobenzoate contrast medium is given as for an IVU, and then X-rays are taken before and after giving several glasses of water or a diuretic such as frusemide. Normally the sudden flow of filtrate that follows the dose of frusemide washes out all the contrast medium from the kidney and ureter within a few minutes but when there is obstruction it accumulates and distends the renal pelvis, and may cause pain in the loin.

The renogram

The same information may be obtained with less irradiation to the patient with a 'diuresis renogram'. Here, a pair of Geiger counters are aimed at the kidneys, and radioactive I 131 Hippuran is given intravenously (Fig. 3. 15) which is filtered and concentrated just like iodobenzoate. As it pools in the dilated renal pelvis the counter registers a climbing curve of radioactivity. At this stage nobody knows whether there is obstruction or just a big floppy renal pelvis, but if the radioactivity goes on rising after frusemide has been given then it means that there is true obstruction (Fig. 3.16).

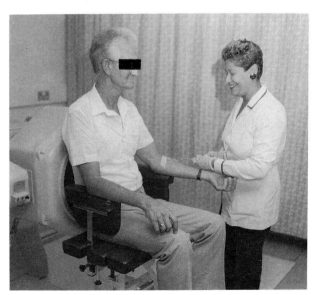

Fig. 3.15 Isotope renogram: the patient sits in front of a gamma camera.

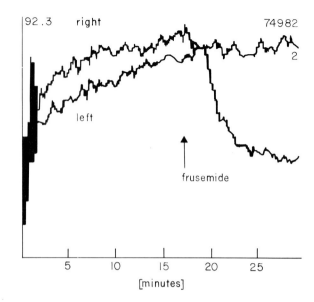

Fig. 3.16 Renogram in a patient with a left-sided obstruction: the curve continues to climb as the isotope accumulates on the obstructed side, while on the unobstructed side it is washed out as soon as frusemide is given.

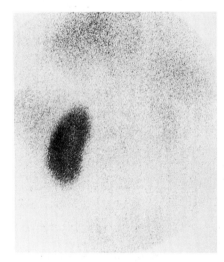

Fig. 3.17 Image of the renal parenchyma provided by the gamma camera after the isotope has been given which is taken up by the renal tubules. Note the missing left kidney.

Most patients find these tests quite interesting and painless although some are a little daunted by the amount of equipment that is involved. The main advantage of isotope renography is that a much smaller dose of radiation is received by the patient than in a IVU.

The gamma camera

Instead of a pair of big Geiger counters a whole battery of very thin ones can be mounted behind the kidney which provides a speckled image of the kidney as it takes up the isotope (Fig. 3.17). The images are less clear than those obtained with an IVU, but much less radiation is needed and they can give more precise information about the functions of the cortex and medulla since one may choose an isotope that is mainly filtered through the glomeruli (DTPA) or one that is secreted by the tubules (DMSA).

The Whitaker test

Even these investigations may fail to make it certain whether the collecting system is obstructed or not. In Whitaker's test the patient lies prone while a fine tube is passed into the renal pelvis with local anaesthetic under X-ray control. Saline can be injected at a rate equal to the maximum possible rate of urine formation (10 ml/s) and the pressure in the tube is recorded. If there is no rise in pressure, obstruction is ruled out (Fig. 3.18).

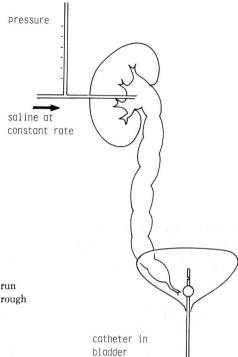

pressure

saline at
constant rate

catheter in
bladder

Fig. 3.18 Whitaker's test: saline is run
into the kidney at a constant rate through
a fine catheter introduced
percutaneously and the pressure is
measured: if it rises, there is
obstruction in the system.

Further reading

Barratt, T. M. (1976) Fundamentals of renal physiology. In *Scientific Foundations of Urology*, eds Williams, D. I. & Chisholm, G. D., pp. 19–27. Heinemann, London.

Britton, K. E. (1985) Radionuclide studies. In *Textbook of Genito-Urinary Surgery*, vol. 1, eds Whitfield, H. N. & Hendry, W. F., pp. 67–103. Churchill Livingstone, Edinburgh.

Hately, W. (1985) Ultrasound investigations of the genito-urinary tract. In *Textbook of Genito-Urinary Surgery*, vol. 1, eds Whitfield, H. N. & Hendry, W. F., pp. 29–52. Churchill Livingstone, Edinburgh.

Haycock, G. B. (1987) Renal function. In *Scientific Basis of Urology*, ed. Mundy, A. R., pp. 1–33. Churchill Livingstone, Edinburgh.

Husband, J. E. & Kellett, M. J. (1985) CT scanning in urology. In *Textbook of Genito-Urinary Surgery*, vol. 1, eds Whitfield, H. N. & Hendry, W. F. pp. 53–66. Churchill Livingstone, Edinburgh.

Lalli, A. F. (1980) Contrast media reactions: data analysis and hypothesis. *Radiology* **134**, 1–12.

Sherwood, T. (1985) Basic uroradiological investigations. In *Textbook of Genito-Urinary Surgery*, vol. 1, eds Whitfield, H. N. & Hendry, W. F., pp. 5–21. Churchill Livingstone, Edinburgh.

4 *The kidney — congenital disorders*

Absence or abnormal position of the kidney

The kidney may be absent on one or other side, sometimes there is neither kidney nor ureter — *agenesis* (Fig. 4.1), sometimes there is a poorly formed ureter but no kidney at all — *aplasia* (Fig. 4.2), sometimes the ureter is almost normal but the kidney is small and malformed — *dysplasia* (Fig. 4.3). These oddities are only important when they lead to infection, obstruction or hypertension. The life expectancy of a patient with only one kidney is just as good as someone with two.

The kidney may lie anywhere along a line between its normal position in the loin right down to alongside the bladder, where it is called a *pelvic kidney* (Fig. 4.4). Pelvic kidneys seldom cause trouble — even in childbirth. They are usually found by accident and seldom need any treatment.

The normal kidney moves up and down with respiration and in some people, especially slim women, the kidney may move from the normal position in the loin right down into the iliac fossa. This, by itself is harmless, but very rarely it is associated with intermittent obstruction to the ureter. These very rare, true examples of *floating* kidney may require

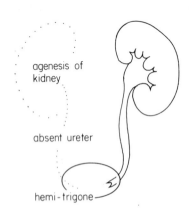

Fig. 4.1 In agenesis of the kidney there is no kidney or ureter at all on one side.

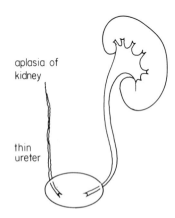

Fig. 4.2 In aplasia there is a thin ureter but no development of a kidney.

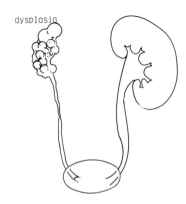

Fig. 4.3 In dysplasia there is a ureter and a kidney, but the kidney is malformed and often tiny and cystic.

an operation to stitch them in position — nephropexy. It must be emphasized that the majority of people in whom this diagnosis is suggested have perfectly normal kidneys and need no treatment at all.

One kidney may get attached to the other in the course of development. If they join in the midline, they form a *horseshoe* kidney (Fig. 4.5). If one wanders across the midline to the other side it is called *crossed renal ectopia* (Fig. 4.6). These conditions would not matter at all except that one congenital anomaly tends to go along with another and there may be coincidental reflux or obstruction at the pelviureteric junction (see p. 109).

Thoracic kidney

In babies with congenital weakness of one half of the diaphragm the abdominal contents may rise into the chest, along with the kidney (Fig. 4.7). Although classified with other types of abnormality in position of a kidney, this is a developmental abnormality of the diaphragm, not the kidney.

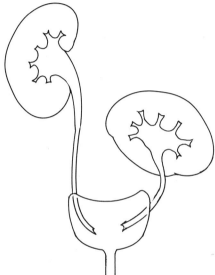

Fig. 4.4 A pelvic kidney may lie in front of the sacrum and be difficult to see.

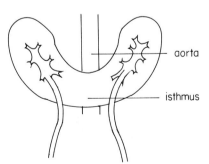

Fig. 4.5 In a horseshoe kidney the two kidneys are joined in the midline in front of the aorta.

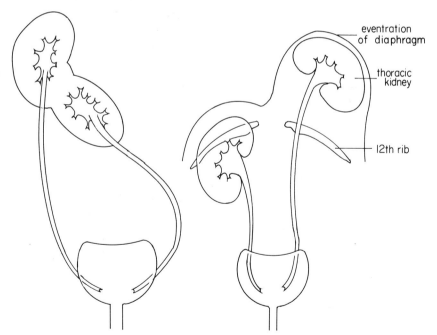

Fig. 4.6 In crossed renal ectopia one kidney crosses over to join the other one.

Fig. 4.7 In so-called thoracic kidney there is a faulty development of the diaphragm which allows the kidney to rise up into the chest.

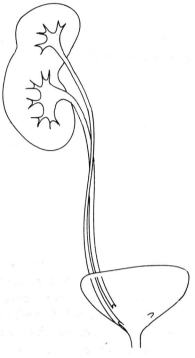

Fig. 4.8 In a duplex kidney the ureter from the upper half-kidney enters the bladder below that from the lower half-kidney.

Duplex kidney

This is a very common anomaly, and usually quite innocent. In the fetus, the kidney begins to form in the pelvis, and on each side a tube — the ureteric bud — sprouts out from what is to become the bladder, to drain the developing kidney. The ureteric bud usually begins to branch when it approaches the kidney to form the renal pelvis and calices but it may begin to divide near the bladder, forming a duplex ureter. Because of the way the ureteric buds are curved, the ureter from the upper part of the kidney enters the bladder a little way below the opening of the ureter from the lower part of the kidney (Fig. 4.8).

Although duplex ureters are common, they only matter when they are associated with other abnormalities, such as reflux, incontinence or ureterocele.

Reflux

The upper of the two ureters may enter the bladder through such a short course that its valve is ineffective, and urine may reflux into the lower half-kidney (Fig. 4.9).

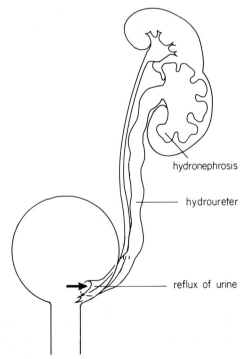

hydronephrosis

hydroureter

reflux of urine

Fig. 4.9 Vesicoureteric reflux allows urine to flow backwards up the upper ureter into the lower half-kidney.

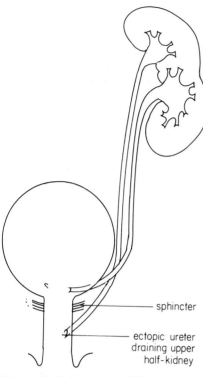

Incontinence

The lower ureter may have such a long tunnel that it enters the urethra downstream of the sphincter and causes incontinence (Fig. 4.10).

Ureterocele

The lower ureter may be covered by a little balloon — a *ureterocele* — which occasionally causes obstruction and sometimes protrudes out of the urethra (Fig. 4.11).

Errors of structure

Cysts of the kidney

Simple cysts can be found in most normal kidneys (Fig. 4.12). Only when they get so big as to cause obstruction to the collecting system do they need treatment but whenever they are detected in a urogram the question is whether this 'space-occupying lesion' is a cancer or a cyst? Nowadays the answer is given by ultrasound or computerized tomography (see p. 25). When there is any doubt a fine needle is passed into the cyst to make sure that its contents are clear of any malignant cells.

Polycystic disease of the kidney is an exaggeration of this condition, but instead of only one or two cysts, the kidney is riddled with them (Fig. 4.13). It occurs in two forms, one inherited, the other not. It may be noticed in childhood but usually the cysts first appear in middle life and get more numerous and more large until, in the end, the kidney is almost

Fig. 4.10 If the more caudally opening ureteric orifice is placed downstream of the sphincter there is persistent leakage of urine — incontinence.

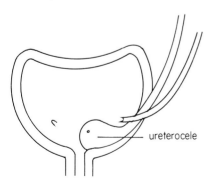

Fig. 4.11 The caudally opening ureteric orifice may open into a balloon-shaped swelling — a ureterocele.

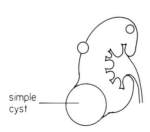

Fig. 4.12 Simple cysts are very common and often found by chance when an ultrasound or a urogram is performed.

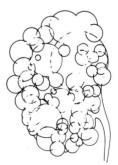

Fig. 4.13 Polycystic kidney: one or both kidneys are riddled with innumerable cysts of different sizes.

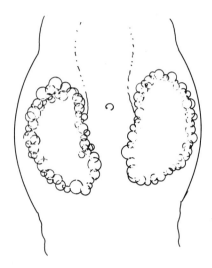

replaced by cysts and renal failure then requires dialysis or transplantation. Occasionally the cysts squeeze the collecting system and have to be deroofed, but this does not improve renal function.

Multicystic disease

In a fetus with obstructed or absent ureters, the nephrons go on making urine until each is converted into a little balloon. If present on one side the baby will have a huge lump which must be removed; if present on both sides there is no medical treatment; perhaps a mercy, since these babies always have many other severe abnormalities; they need tender loving care for the remainder of their brief lives (Fig. 4.14).

Medullary sponge kidney

This is a curious inherited condition associated with hemihypertrophy of the body, i.e. the arm and leg on one side are bigger than the other. The collecting tubules are big and baggy and the urine in them is stagnant, easily infected and forms multiple little stones (Fig. 4.15). The condition may affect one small part of one kidney or all of both of them. It is sometimes inherited and tends to get slowly worse, until eventually the medulla of the kidney is converted into a spongy mass with innumerable stones in

Fig. 4.14 Multicystic disease of the kidneys: the ureters are blocked or absent and one or both kidneys are converted into large collections of cysts.

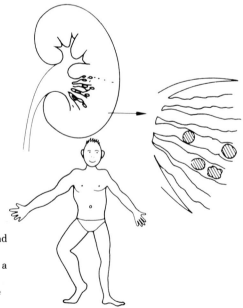

Fig. 4.15 In medullary sponge kidney the collecting tubules become dilated and stones form inside them. Gradually the medulla of the kidney is converted into a swollen spongy mass. The condition is associated with hemihypertrophy of the limbs.

the dilated tubules. The patients have persistent infection and repeated episodes of ureteric colic. If the process is confined to one or two pyramids, they can be removed by a *partial nephrectomy*, but when both kidneys are affected all one can do is to remove stones when they cause obstruction, and try to keep the infection under control. The new techniques of extracorporeal lithotripsy have revolutionized the treatment of this condition.

Further reading

Frank, J. D. (1987) Developmental abnormalities of the urinary tract. In *Scientific Basis of Urology*, ed. Mundy, A. R., pp. 74–91. Churchill Livingstone, Edinburgh.

Johnston, J. H. (1976) Congenital anomalies of the kidney. In *Urology*, vol. 1, ed. Blandy, J. P., pp. 138–153. Blackwell Scientific Publications, Oxford.

Pitts, W. R. & Muecke, E. C. (1975) Horseshoe kidney: a 40 year experience. *Journal of Urology*, **113**, 743–746.

Roback, H. B. (1984) Helping patients and their families cope with medical problems. In *Coping with the Death of a Newborn*, ed. Walwork, E. pp. 409–427. Jossey-Bass, London.

Smith, P. J. B. (1984) Congenital disorders of the kidney. In *Textbook of Genito-Urinary Surgery*, vol. 1, eds Whitfield, H. N. & Hendry W. F. pp. 139–149. Churchill Livingstone, Edinburgh.

Steg, A (1976) Renal cysts. I. Current pathogenic approach. *European Urology*, **2**, 161–163.

5 *The kidney — trauma*

Penetrating wounds

If the kidney is injured by a knife or low-velocity bullet, the penetrating wound will demand surgical exploration, at which the laceration can sometimes be repaired, or a detached fragment of kidney removed.

If the injury has been caused by a modern high-velocity bullet the kidney will be beyond repair and must be removed. Obviously these are grave emergencies requiring intensive resuscitation and massive blood transfusion.

Closed injury of the kidney

In sport and everyday accidents a more or less severe blow to the loin may cause renal injury with fracture of the lower ribs and the transverse processes of the lumbar vertebrae (Fig. 5.1). The kidney is split, and blood leaks into the collecting system to cause haematuria.

The kidney is surrounded by a packing of fat inside a strong thin envelope like a plastic bag — *Gerota's fascia.* Bleeding from the cortex of the kidney fills up Gerota's fascia until it is tight and the kidney stops

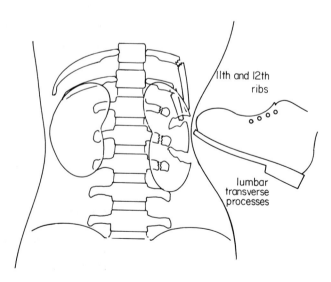

Fig. 5.1 The blunt injury to the loin that leads to rupture of the kidney may also fracture the lower ribs and transverse processes of the lumbar vertebrae.

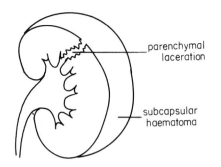

Fig. 5.2 The blood is confined within Gerota's fascia so tightly that the bleeding usually stops spontaneously.

bleeding (Fig. 5.2), so that nearly all closed injuries of the kidney recover without surgical intervention. Very rarely is the bleeding so profuse as to burst Gerota's fascia but since at first it is impossible to predict this rare, unlucky outcome, all these patients are admitted for careful observation.

As soon as possible, an IVU is performed to make sure that there is a kidney on the other side, for if the patient is one of the few who continue to bleed, and needs to be operated on, the only way to stop the haemorrhage may be to remove the kidney.

Blood is taken for grouping and cross-matching.

Conservative management

1 Rest in bed.
2 The pulse rate and blood pressure are recorded every 30 minutes.
3 The abdominal girth is measured hourly to detect any enlargement that might suggest continued bleeding around the kidney.
4 Each specimen of urine is saved, and the time it was passed is marked on the container. If all is going well there will be less and less blood in successive specimens.
5 A high fluid intake is kept up, if necessary, with intravenous fluids.

If there is evidence of internal bleeding, e.g. a swelling in the loin, a rise in pulse rate and a fall in blood pressure — the patient will have an angiogram performed (see p. 27).

The angiogram not only shows just where the kidney has been torn, but it may actually identify the branch of the renal artery which is bleeding and allow the radiologist to seal it off by injecting a plug of muscle or gelfoam (Fig. 5.3). Very rarely the internal haemorrhage is so severe that the patient must be rushed to the operating theatre and then it is hardly ever possible to save the kidney.

Fig. 5.3 If there is continuing haemorrhage from a torn segmental artery it may be possible to plug the artery with gelfoam injected at the time of arteriography.

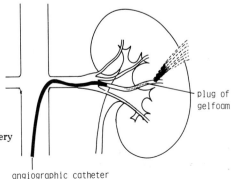

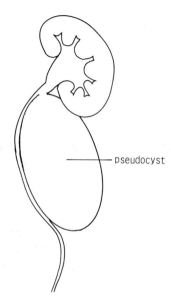

pseudocyst

Fig. 5.4 Rarely there is a collection of urine (urinoma) outside the kidney which forms a pseudocyst that may subsequently become infected and need to be drained or removed.

Although most of these patients recover without the need for anything more than simple rest and observation, there is always a slight risk of secondary haemorrhage, and they should all be kept under observation for about 10 days after the initial injury. During this time it is usual to give antibiotics in case there is any underlying infection in the urinary tract that might infect the haematoma.

A second IVU is performed after 6 weeks and a further one at 1 year to make sure that the kidney is healed. Occasionally this reveals a *hydronephrosis* or a collection of urine outside the kidney — a *urinoma or pseudocyst* which requires surgical correction (Fig. 5.4).

Further reading

Bernath, A. S., Schutte, H., Fernandez, R. R. D. & Addonizio, J. C. (1983) Stab wounds of the kidney — conservative management in flank penetration. *Journal of Urology*, **129**, 468–470.

Conrad, M. R., Freedman, M., Weinger, C., Freeman, C. & Sanders, R. C. (1976) Sonography of the Page kidney. *Journal of Urology*, **116**, 293–296.

Lipsky, H., Petritsch, P. & Schreyer, H. (1975) The role of angiography in diagnosis and management of blunt renal trauma. *British Journal of Urology*, **47**, 711–720.

Mogenson, P., Agger, P. & Ostergaard, A. H. (1980) A conservative approach to the management of blunt renal trauma. *British Journal of Urology*, **52**, 338–341.

Selikowitz, S. M. (1977) Penetrating high-velocity genitourinary injuries. *Urology*, **9**, 371–376.

Thompson, I. M., Ross, G. Jr, Essard J., Habib, H. & Amoury R. A. (1976) Experiences with 16 cases of pararenal pseudocyst. *Journal of Urology*, **116**, 289–292.

6 *The kidney — inflammations*

There are two main types of inflammatory disease of the kidney — those caused by allergy, which affect the glomerulus, *glomerulonephritis*; and those caused by bacteria, which affect the collecting system, *pyelonephritis*.

Glomerulonephritis

When antigen-antibody complexes of many kinds settle on the glomerular filter they may damage it and as a result, larger particles escape along with the solutes of the normal glomerular filtrate. When the damage is slight, only plasma proteins can leak out, but so much may be lost that the plasma proteins become depleted and unable to retain the water in the blood stream from seeping out into the tissues as oedema and ascites. The resulting combination of widespread oedema, ascites and proteinuria is called the *nephrotic syndrome*.

If the damage to the glomerular filter is more severe red cells as well as protein leak through it giving rise to haematuria, sometimes enough to block up the tubules and lead to oliguria, renal failure and hypertension — the *nephritic syndrome*. The nursing care of this important group of diseases is beyond the scope of this book, but is dealt with in textbooks on medical renal disorders.

Pyelonephritis

A major part of urological diagnosis and treatment is aimed at preventing damage to the kidneys from bacterial infection.

Ascending infection

Urine is an excellent culture medium for any bacteria (in fact Pasteur used urine in his historical experiments). When bacteria reach the collecting system they cause acute inflammation and the lining of the ureter, renal pelvis and calices becomes red, painful and swollen.

This is pyelonephritis: the kidney is acutely painful, there are pus cells and bacteria in the urine and the patient may be very ill with a high fever, But the name covers two distinct conditions, one merely a nuisance, the other potentially dangerous.

When the inflammation is limited to the epithelium that lines the collecting system — as it is in many patients whose urinary infection is accompanied by pain in the loin and fever — it resolves without any aftermath. But when the bacteria penetrate deep into the kidney tissue the inflammation that results may have much more serious consequences. This occurs by *intrarenal reflux* when an increased pressure inside the collecting system forces infected urine back up the collecting tubules into the renal pyramid (Fig. 6.1). The resulting interstitial inflammation of the renal medulla causes fever and pain in the loin, and when severe the swelling may even prevent urine getting out of the affected pyramids of the kidney. There are three possible results:

1 Resolution, when everything returns to normal.

2 Scarring, when healing is followed by deeply pitted contracted scars in the kidney cortex.

3 Papillary necrosis — one or more renal papillae containing the stems of the collecting tubules and the long loops of Henle may die and ultimately separate into the renal pelvis (Fig. 6.2).

These more serious results of the combination of back pressure and infection occur most often in children with vesicoureteric reflux, but may also be seen after almost any combination of obstruction and infection.

Reflux nephropathy

In babies, a congenitally incompetent valve at the entry of the ureters into the bladder allows *vesicoureteric reflux* so that urine is forced back from the bladder to the kidney. In some of these babies there is an additional deformity of the renal papillae. Normally the collecting ducts open

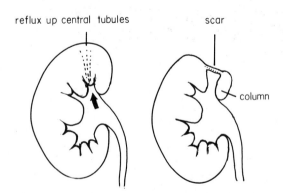

Fig. 6.1 Bacteria carried by intrarenal reflux into the cortex give rise to inflammation that may be followed by the formation of a typical pitted scar.

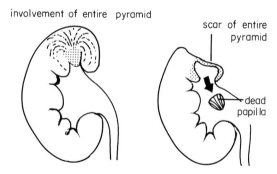

Fig. 6.2 In severe infections the whole pyramid may be involved and the renal papilla may die off (papillary necrosis).

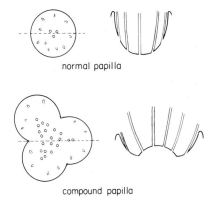

normal papilla

compound papilla

Fig. 6.3 Some children are born with malformed (compound) papillae which have an ineffective valve and readily allow intrarenal reflux of urine to occur.

obliquely on the sides of the papilla and intra-renal reflux is prevented by their valvular action, but when the papillae are clustered together the ducts open on the middle of a crater, and there is no protective valve to prevent intrarenal reflux of infected urine (Fig. 6.3).

Vesicoureteric reflux is detected by means of a *micturating cystogram* (Fig. 6.4). Contrast medium is put into the bladder through a fine catheter and X-rays are taken while the baby passes water which show the urine going back up the ureters, and even entering the pyramids. For this investigation parental consent is of course required and some sedation may be necessary.

Reflux pyelonephritis in children can lead to devastating and irreversible scarring of the kidney, and the damage has often been done by the time the condition is first detected. If infection can be kept under control by antibiotics the condition may be prevented from worsening, but if it cannot be controlled it is necessary to reimplant the ureters in such a way as to prevent reflux.

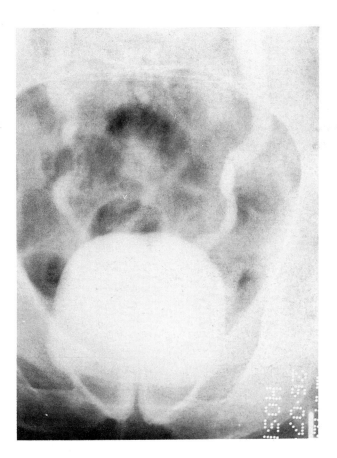

Fig. 6.4 A micturating cystogram showing reflux of urine from the bladder up both ureters.

There are several alternative methods of making this new valve. Most of them require an operation at which the ureter is dissected free and drawn under a new submucosal tunnel in the bladder (Fig. 6.5). Recently it is claimed that the same result may be achieved by injecting a tiny blob of Teflon paste under the ureteric orifice through a cystoscope (Fig. 6.6).

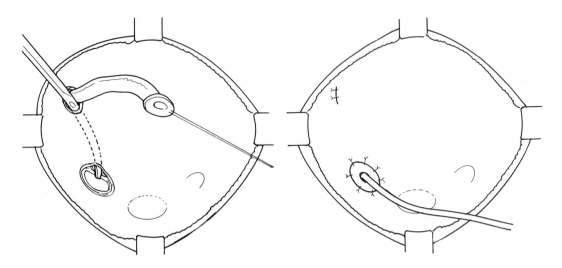

Fig. 6.5 Leadbetter-Politano operation for re-implantation of ureter to correct vesicoureteric reflux.

Other types of obstructive uropathy

Very similar intrarenal reflux of infected urine followed by scarring of the pyramid and loss of the papilla may be seen at any age when there is infection accompanied by obstruction e.g. from a stone. Obstruction alone causes a less vicious effect on the kidney: it slowly erodes the papillae, but does not have the added damage that follows the entry of infected urine into the renal tissue. In uninfected obstruction the renal medulla suffers most, but glomerular filtration may be hardly affected, and the kidney continues to secrete large volumes of unconcentrated urine which can lead to dehydration and salt loss.

Septicaemia and septicaemic shock

This may occur after any urological procedure from the most trivial — passing or removing a catheter — to the most major surgery, because the urinary tract is lined by such very delicate epithelium that it is easy for microorganisms to gain entry to the blood stream when this epithelium is scratched or torn.

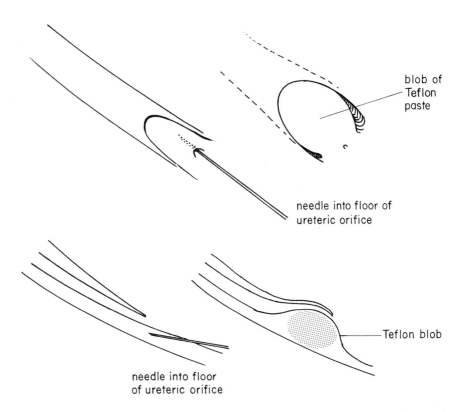

blob of
Teflon
paste

needle into floor of
ureteric orifice

needle into floor
of ureteric orifice

Teflon blob

Fig. 6.6 Reflux may be prevented by injecting a small blob of Teflon paste under the ureteric orifice through a cystoscope.

As a result a sharp look out must be kept for septicaemia in all urological patients. The danger is most in those who have the combination of obstruction and infected urine because the infected urine can so easily enter the lymphatics of the kidney (Fig. 6.7).

The first warning sign is usually a rigor. The patient shivers uncontrollably and says he feels cold. He has a rapid pulse, rising temperature, and a falling blood pressure. He becomes restless and hot and may complain of headache. At this stage he looks red and his skin is warm due to the peripheral vasodilatation; he is often confused. It is most important that these warning signs are recognized for there is no time to lose if a life is to be saved. Delay may allow the patient to slide into irreversible and fatal septicaemic shock.

Three emergency measures must be taken:

1 *The diagnosis must be confirmed.* There may be other causes for shock in these surgical patients. One must make sure there has been no unexpected haemorrhage and an electrocardiogram is taken to rule out a myocardial infarction.

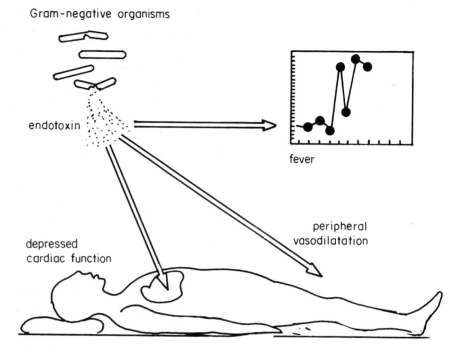

Gram-negative organisms

endotoxin

fever

peripheral vasodilatation

depressed cardiac function

Fig. 6.7 The changes of septicaemic shock.

2 *The bacteria must be killed.* Blood is taken for culture, and sent to the laboratory at once. Massive doses of bactericidal drugs are given. Often it is only possible to guess which drug to use unless it is known which microorganisms are already present in the urine. If the preoperative urine was sterile, the infection will probably have been acquired in hospital, and the hospital laboratory will know which organisms are most likely to be the cause of cross-infection and can advise as to the most effective antibiotics to use.

3 *Blood volume must be replaced.* An intravenous infusion is set up. During the phase of septicaemia the patient has too little blood to fill the dilated peripheral blood vessels and a large infusion of blood, plasma or haemacel is occasionally needed. Up to 5 or 6 litres may have to be given in the first few hours in order to maintain the blood pressure and a *central venous pressure line* may be necessary to monitor the pressure in the right atrium and make sure that the patient is not overloaded (Fig. 6.7).

If these emergency measures are taken promptly, the patient usually recovers. Within hours the peripheral blood vessels regain their tone and the myocardium recovers from its brief episode of poisoning. Now the patient may become overloaded with fluid and oedema of the lungs may make him short of breath. Usually the kidneys get rid of this excess of fluid in the urine but it may be necessary to give a diuretic intravenously to hasten this process and sometimes it may be necessary to remove one or two pints of blood by *venesection* — storing it to be given back later.

If these measures are not taken in time the patient remains in shock. He becomes increasingly oedematous and there is a progressive impairment of oxygen exchange in the lungs. There also follows an alteration in the coagulating system of the blood (disseminated intravascular coagulation or DIC) that leads to renal failure and makes the lung infection even worse, and despite every care, the patient dies.

Even when treatment seems to be working, continuous, careful observation of the patient must be kept up throughout all these changes: temperature, pulse, respiration and blood pressure must be recorded every half hour until the condition is at last stable. By this time the patient will probably have perspired profusely, and will appreciate a wash and a change of clothes.

The sudden onset of septicaemic shock: the speed with which the patient changes from being hot, red and agitated into a state of profound shock; and the rapidity of the recovery when chemotherapy and fluids are given, makes this a most dramatic condition to manage. Nurses need to be alert to the warning signs that things may be going wrong.

To avoid the danger of septicaemia *prophylactic antibiotics* are usually given to patients with known infection in their urine before any urological procedure.

Analgesic nephropathy

Other things cause damage to the kidney very similar to that which is caused by bacteria, i.e. scarring of the renal pyramid and sloughing of the papillae. One of the most important is *analgesic nephropathy*. People may consume large amounts of analgesics such as aspirins, phenacitin and codeine day in and day out, sometimes because of pain from rheumatism, more often from bad habit. This leads to a vicious cycle: when they stop taking analgesics a headache develops, and so they have to take more and so on. The kidney becomes scarred, the papillae may die and fall off into the renal collecting system blocking it just like a stone. (Fig. 6.8).

Balkan nephropathy

Along the valley of the Danube where farmers store grain in damp barns, people are poisoned by a toxin that is thought to be produced by a mould. It causes progressive scarring in the kidneys and necrosis of the renal papillae.

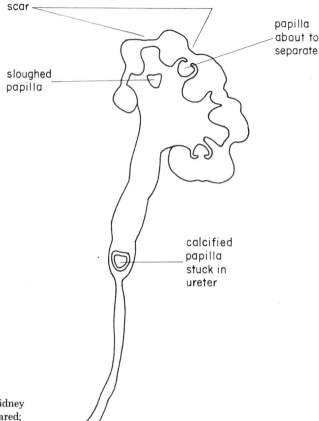

scar

papilla
about to
separate

sloughed
papilla

calcified
papilla
stuck in
ureter

Fig. 6.8 The end stage of analgesic nephropathy: the kidney is deeply pitted and scarred; some papillae have disappeared; others are partially separated; one is stuck in the ureter.

Renal tuberculosis

The kidney is always infected via the blood stream from a distant primary focus, generally in the lung, which has been dormant for years. In the kidneys the disease starts as a little abscess in a renal papilla which is at first symptomless, until it bursts into the collecting system. Now irritating debris is carried down the ureter to the bladder, giving rise to discomfort and frequency of urination. By the time it is first diagnosed, there is always some erosion of the renal papillae, or the late changes of *caseation* where a confluent mass of tuberculous abscesses has converted most of the kidney into something resembling cottage cheese (Fig. 6.9).

The diagnosis of tuberculosis in the urinary tract is always difficult because the organisms are scanty and difficult to grow in the laboratory. It is suspected whenever there are pus cells in the urine that seem to grow no organism — *sterile pyuria*. The tubercle bacilli may be found in the urine

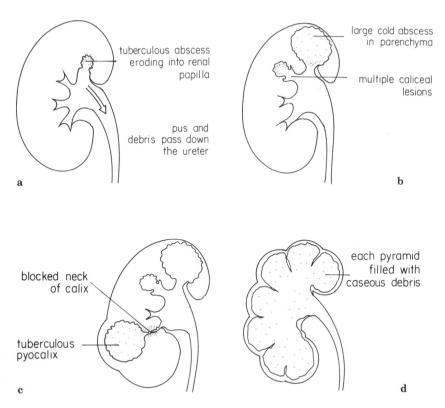

Fig. 6.9 The progress of tuberculosis in the kidney from the first small lesion in a papilla (a) to the complete replacement of the kidney by a bag of caseous tissue — the 'cement kidney' (b).

using a stain which becomes fixed in the waxy envelope of the tubercle bacilli, and cannot be washed out with acid or alcohol (hence the name acid-fast bacilli or AFB). But other particles, notably sperms, take up this stain and to avoid mistakes the diagnosis must be confirmed by culture — a process which takes 6 weeks, and is done using collections of three specimens of all the urine passed in the morning (early morning urine or 'EMU × 3').

Nowadays with prompt chemotherapy, patients with genitourinary tuberculosis are usually cured within months. But they all have to be followed very carefully during the first few weeks after treatment has started because there are often unsuspected patches of tuberculosis in the ureter or the wall of the bladder. As the chemotherapy kills off the tubercle bacilli, their nesting places are replaced with scar tissue, and these scars contract, so that the ureter can become so narrow that it leads to obstruction, and the wall of the bladder may shrink so much that its capacity is no more than that of an egg-cup (Fig. 6.10).

A narrowing at the upper end of the ureter can be corrected by a pyeloplasty (see p. 109) and at the lower end by being reimplanted into the bladder (see p. 47). When the bladder is contracted patients may have so much frequency and discomfort that it has to be enlarged. The usual method is to add on an isolated segment of caecum (see caecocystoplasty, p. 152).

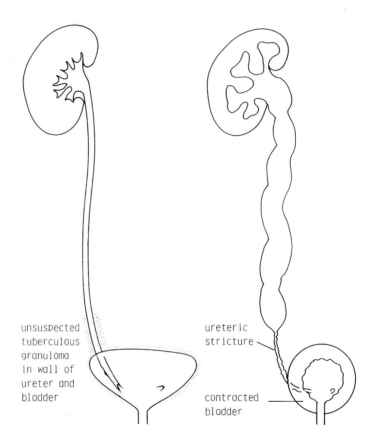

Fig. 6.10 Rapid healing follows chemotherapy for tuberculosis, and in the wall of the ureter and bladder the scars quickly contract.

Malakoplakia and xanthogranuloma

These are rare but exceedingly dangerous chronic inflammations of the kidney which start off as infections with *Escherichia coli* and *Proteus mirabilis*, usually associated with a stone. Instead of a small scarred kidney, they produce a stiff honeycomb of abscesses. The patient has a continual fever, develops fistulae and sinuses, and loses weight. It may be difficult to distinguish such a chronic granuloma from cancer of the kidney. Treatment has to be equally aggressive for even though this is a benign disease it does not respond to antibiotics and unless surgically excised will prove fatal.

Hydatid disease of the kidney

Dogs that eat meat from sheep infected with the tapeworm *Echinococcus granulosus* grow the worm in their intestine. Its eggs are passed in the dog's faeces onto its fur, from which they reach the hands of the owners or their children and are accidentally eaten. Hatching inside the intestine the larvae bore through the stomach, and are carried in the portal vein to the liver, where they usually remain. Occasionally a few are carried round the circulation to other organs, including the kidney.

In the kidney they settle down and grow into collections of cysts containing a watery fluid, hence the name — *hydatid cysts* (Fig. 6.11). These hydatid cysts are the breeding places for hundreds of tiny tapeworms — *scolices*. Just as an oyster surrounds a grain of sand with a shell of pearl, so the patient surrounds the hydatid cysts by a wall of calcified fibrous tissue. In the IVU and ultrasound these multiple calcified cysts can look like cancer. The cysts are translucent on ultrasound, and serological tests may be needed to confirm the diagnosis. Nephrectomy is the usual treatment. Before a collection of cysts is removed it is necessary to kill off the tiny tapeworms inside by aspirating the fluid and replacing it with hypertonic saline, 2.5% formalin or 0.5% silver nitrate. Unless this precaution is taken, the tiny tapeworms may be scattered at operation throughout the tissues, with massive local recurrences that are usually fatal. There is at present no reliable chemotherapy for hydatid disease.

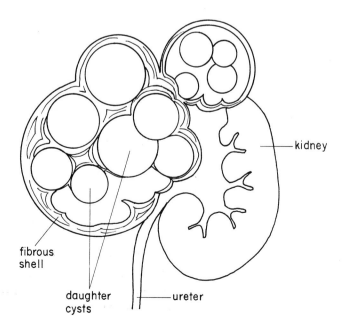

Fig. 6.11 Hydatid cysts in the kidney.

Cortical abscess and renal carbuncle

In diabetics and others with poor resistance, blood-borne infection, usually with *Staphylococcus aureus*, may get to the kidney and settle in the cortex to form a *parenchymal abscess* (Fig. 6.12) which is outside the collecting system, so there are no pus cells or bacteria in the urine, but the patient is ill with a tender swollen kidney and a fever. The IVU shows a soft tissue mass that resembles cancer, but ultrasound and CT scans show that the mass has the consistency of pus, not cancer, and the diagnosis can be confirmed by aspirating pus with a needle and syringe.

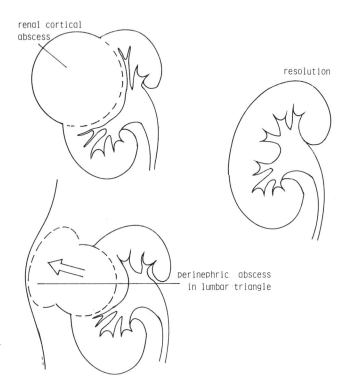

Fig. 6.12 A cortical abscess usually resolves with antibiotic treatment but may burst through the renal capsule to form a perinephric abscess.

Explain to the patient that there is a collection of pus in the loin, and that this can be sucked out with a needle, which will be put in after the track has been made numb with a local anaesthetic. The abscess is located with ultrasound. Local anaesthetic is injected with a very fine needle along the track leading to the abscess until aspiration on the syringe yields pus. A larger needle is then passed along the anaesthetized track to empty the abscess completely. The pus is sent for culture and sensitivity. Guided by this information from the laboratory, an intensive course of antibiotics is then given, and the mass usually disappears — a process which today can be checked by repeated ultrasound examinations.

Further reading

Birmingham Reflux Study Group (1983) Prospective trial of operative versus non-operative treatment of severe vesicoureteric reflux: two years observation in 96 children. *British Medical Journal*, **287**, 171–174.

Blandy, J. P. (1976) Surgical infections of the kidney. In *Urology*, vol. 1, ed. Blandy, J. P., pp. 195–225. Blackwell Scientific Publications, Oxford.

Casewell, M. (1979) Bacteria danger on the ward. *Nursing Mirror*, May 17, 37–39.

Cooke, N. J. (1985) Treatment of tuberculosis. *British Medical Journal*, **291**, 497.

Cowie, A. G. A. (1985) Parasitic infections. In *Textbook of Genito-Urinary Surgery*, eds Whitfield, H. N. & Hendry, W. F. pp. 536–546. Churchill Livingstone, Edinburgh.

Flynn, J. T., Molland, E. A., Paris, A. M. I. & Blandy, J. P. (1979) The underestimated hazards of xanthogranulomatous pyelonephritis. *British Journal of Urology*, **51**, 443–445.

Gow, J. G. (1984) Genito-urinary tuberculosis. In *Textbook of Genito-Urinary Surgery*, vol. 1, eds Whitfield, H. N. & Hendry, W. F., pp. 546–555. Churchill Livingstone, Edinburgh.

Gow, J. G. & Barbosa, S. (1984) Genitourinary tuberculosis: a study of 1117 cases over a period of 34 years. *British Journal of Urology*, **56**, 449–455.

Kincaid-Smith, P. (1983) Reflux nephropathy. *British Medical Journal*, **286**, 2002–2003.

Lambert, H. P. (1985) Septicaemia associated with the genito-urinary tract. In *Textbook of Genito-Urinary Surgery*, vol. 1, eds Whitfield, H. N. & Hendry, W. F., pp. 518–523. Churchill Livingstone, Edinburgh.

McKerrow, W., Davidson-Lamb, N. & Jones, P. F. (1984) Urinary tract infection in children. *British Medical Journal*, **289**, 299–303.

Puri, P. & O'Donnell, B. (1984) Correction of experimentally produced vesicoureteric reflux in the piglet by intravesical injection of Teflon. *British Medical Journal*, **289**, 5–10.

Saidi, F. (1976) *Surgery of Hydatid Disease*. Saunders, London. Smellie, J. M., Ransley, P. G., Normand, I. C. S., Prescod, N. & Edwards, D. (1985) Development of new renal scars: a collaborative study. *British Medical Journal*, **290**, 1957–1959.

7 *The kidney — cancer*

Wilms' tumour of children

This occurs in children under the age of 6. They have pain, a swelling in the abdomen, and sometimes blood in the urine. Ultrasound and urography show a large mass deforming the kidney (Fig. 7.1). Until recently this was lethal but nowadays almost every child can be cured by a combination of surgical excision of the tumour and chemotherapy with actinomycin D and vincristine which deal with the microscopical remnants of the tumour that are beyond the limits of surgical resection.

To get the best results in this rare tumour all these children should be referred to centres where the dose and choice of chemotherapy, and the correct sequence of surgery and radiotherapy are under constant audit and continually improved.

Grawitz tumour of adults

Although more common in elderly men, this tumour can occur in either sex and at any age. Unsuspected for many years, it is usually only noticed

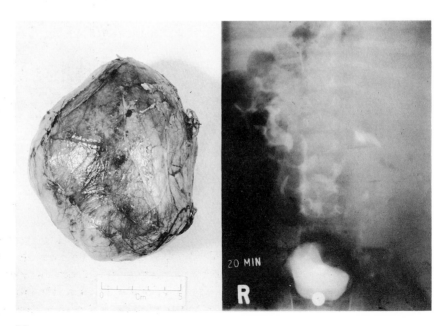

Fig. 7.1 A Wilms' tumour removed by operation — note the relatively large size of the mass compared with the size of the baby.

when it is very large, and gives rise to haematuria, a lump and occasionally pain. An IVU shows a large space-occupying lesion distorting the calices. Ultrasound shows that the lesion is solid rather than cystic. If in doubt an angiogram will confirm the diagnosis by revealing the typically rich blood supply of a cancer of the kidney (Fig. 7.2).

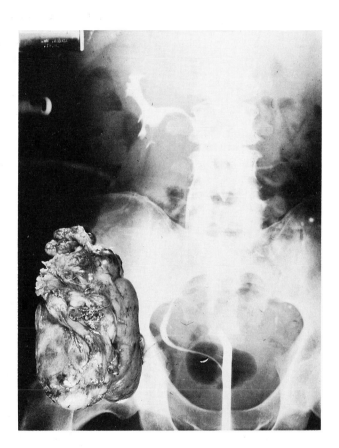

Fig. 7.2 The pyelogram and operative specimen of an adenocarcinoma of the kidney in an adult (Grawitz tumour).

Renal carcinoma grows into the renal vein and tumour cells are easily carried off in the vena cava via the heart to the lungs where they settle and grow into rounded lumps of secondary cancer — 'cannon-ball' metastases.

For most tumours the treatment is *radical nephrectomy* which is sometimes preceded by embolization of the whole kidney to reduce bleeding at the time of operation (see p. 27). This is done 24 to 48 hours before surgery. It may cause considerable pain needing strong analgesia. Very occasionally in small tumours, and in tumours occurring simultaneously in both kidneys, a partial nephrectomy will be performed.

Radical nephrectomy

This procedure is carried out when the tumour is very vascular with a lump of tumour in the renal vein that encroaches on the vena cava. Some surgeons approach them from the front — the *transabdominal approach*, others prefer a *thoraco-abdominal* incision. Whatever the route a big incision is needed if the operation is to be safe as well as radical.

The colon and duodenum are lifted off the front of the kidney. A ligature is placed around the renal artery to cut off the blood supply to the mass and prevent loss of blood during the rest of the dissection. Then the renal vein is divided. Sometimes the vena cava must be opened to remove tumour from its lumen. Finally the ureter is divided and the mass removed (Figs 7.3 and 7.4).

Nursing care

The patient must be prepared for the loss of a kidney, a painful incision, the possibility of an underwater sealed chest drain, a urethral catheter, blood transfusion and a period of paralytic ileus.

When nephrectomy is required, patients must be reassured that they can lead a normal life with only one kidney, indeed, the life expectancy for a patient with only one kidney is just as good as for someone with two — and it can be a great comfort to repeat this well-documented statistic. The operation is seldom done when there is doubt about the function of the good kidney, and in such cases care is taken to make sure that dialysis is possible.

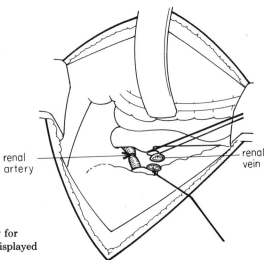

renal artery

renal vein

Fig. 7.3 In radical nephrectomy for renal cancer the renal artery is displayed and ligated before the vein.

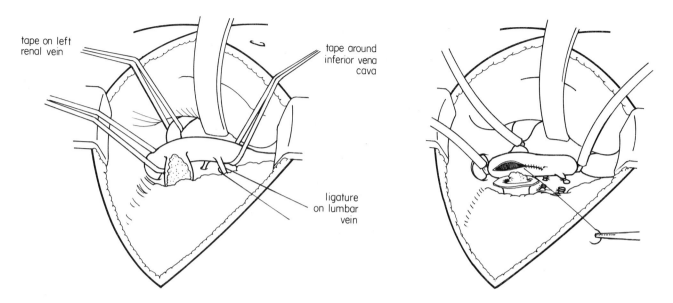

Fig. 7.4 Tumour in the renal vein may protrude into the inferior vena cava; the veins are taped to control bleeding before the lump is removed from the vena cava.

In view of the big incision, sometimes a transthoracic one, and the risk of postoperative pulmonary complications, breathing exercises under the supervision of a physiotherapist are useful both before and after the operation, along with the assurance that adequate analgesia will be available when it is needed. If a chest drain has been used it will remain for one or two days until the lung remains fully expanded.

These tumours are very vascular and large volumes of blood may be needed. Should the blood pressure fall, there is a risk to the remaining kidney so the output of urine is monitored carefully via a urethral catheter. Enough intravenous fluids are given to ensure an output of about 50 ml urine per hour in the early postoperative period. The catheter remains in position until the patient's condition is stable and he or she can cooperate in passing urine. Intravenous therapy is continued until postoperative ileus is over and oral fluids are tolerated in normal amounts. Food may be taken as the appetite returns.

Everyone must be alert to the possibility of postoperative reactionary haemorrhage from vessels in the muscular wall of the abdomen which may need the application of a firm dressing. Deep vein thrombosis is always a hazard, as after any major operation, and perhaps pulmonary embolism is more common when the vena cava has had to be opened. Moving the patient's position, exercising the legs at least every 2 hours while he is in bed, and mobilization as soon as the general condition permits reduce the risk of this complication.

If all goes smoothly the patient should be home within 2 weeks, and able to resume normal activities after 6 weeks.

Adjuvant therapy

In contrast to the Wilms' tumour of children, neither radiotherapy nor chemotherapy has been of any use as an adjuvant to nephrectomy for carcinoma of the kidney in adults, but radiotherapy has a limited place in the treatment of localized painful metastases.

Cancer of the kidney is a very unusual tumour. We hardly ever see a patient with a small one; nearly always they are very large before metastases appear, suggesting that the body has an effective way of fighting this particular cancer. Many patients present with fever, loss of weight and a raised sedimentation rate — suggesting that their immune defence systems are trying to combat the growth.

Metastases sometimes disappear if the primary tumour is removed; this is rare but it raises the hope that maybe one day it will be possible to stimulate these natural body defences.

The prognosis is always uncertain, but never altogether gloomy and even when metastases appear many years after the removal of the primary tumour, they can be treated and the patient may still have many more years of life.

Cancer of the collecting system

Urothelial cancer affects any part of the collecting system from the renal calices all the way down to the urethra and it may occur simultaneously in several parts at the same time. Predisposing factors are analgesic abuse, Balkan nephropathy, smoking, and exposure to industrial carcinogens in the chemical, dyestuffs and rubber industries. It causes haematuria, sometimes so heavy as to cause colic when clots are passed down the ureter.

Urine cytology

The diagnosis may be made by finding malignant cells in the urine (Fig. 7.5). For this purpose urine voided in the daytime — rather than the stale urine passed first thing in the morning — is best. The cells are preserved by adding a fixative such as 10% formalin solution (in roughly an equal volume). The fixed urine is centrifuged in the laboratory, and the deposit is stained and examined for malignant cells using stains introduced by Papanicolaou.

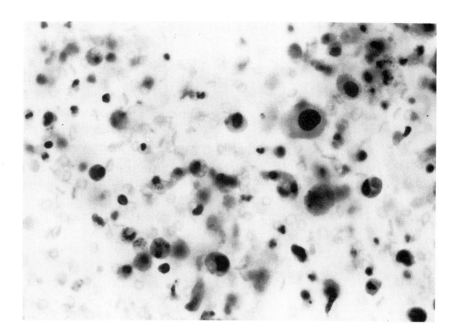

Fig. 7.5 Urothelial cancer cells in urine.

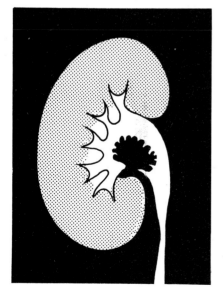

Fig. 7.6 A urogram may show a filling defect due to a carcinoma in the renal pelvis.

Urography

The IVU may show a filling defect in the renal pelvis or ureter (Fig. 7.6). Cystoscopy is needed to rule out coincidental cancer in the bladder. A ureteric catheter is passed into the ureteric orifice and contrast medium is injected to obtain a *retrograde urogram* which will show tumours in the pelvis and ureter as filling defects.

A fine catheter with a little brush on the end (Fig. 7.7) may be passed into the renal pelvis under X-ray control. It is rubbed against the filling defect to collect cancer cells. The brush is removed, cut off, and dropped into formalin. In the laboratory the cells are shaken from the brush with an ultrasonic vibrator, centrifuged, and stained by Papanicolaou's method.

A rigid *ureteroscope* (Fig. 7.8) may be passed up the ureter to give a view of the tumour and allow a direct biopsy to be taken with a forceps and possibly laser treatment. To know the histology of the growth can be important. These tumours come in three grades of malignancy (G1, G2 and G3). In the worst grade, G3, a course of radiotherapy is often given before surgical excision. In the good grade 1 some tumours can be removed by local excision without taking away the kidney or the ureter but unfortunately such good tumours are the exception and the usual treatment is radical *nephroureterectomy*.

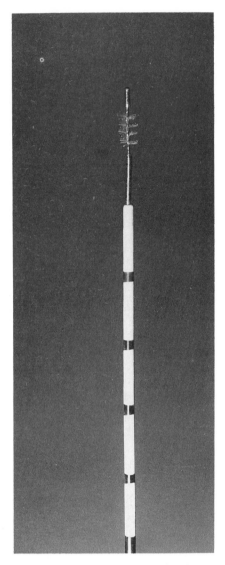

Fig. 7.7 Ureteric catheter with brush to obtain cells from a tumour in the renal pelvis or ureter.

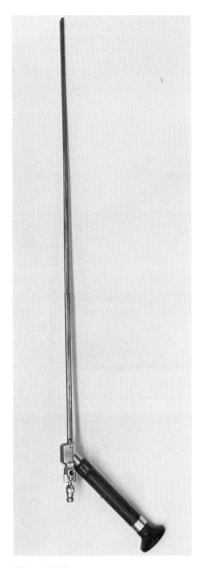

Fig. 7.8 Ureteroscope.

Nephroureterectomy

The kidney is removed with all its surrounding fat and connective tissue to avoid spilling any growth in the wound (Fig. 7.9). Then, through a second incision, the bladder is opened, and the lower end of the ureter removed together with an ellipse of surrounding bladder (Fig. 7.10). The

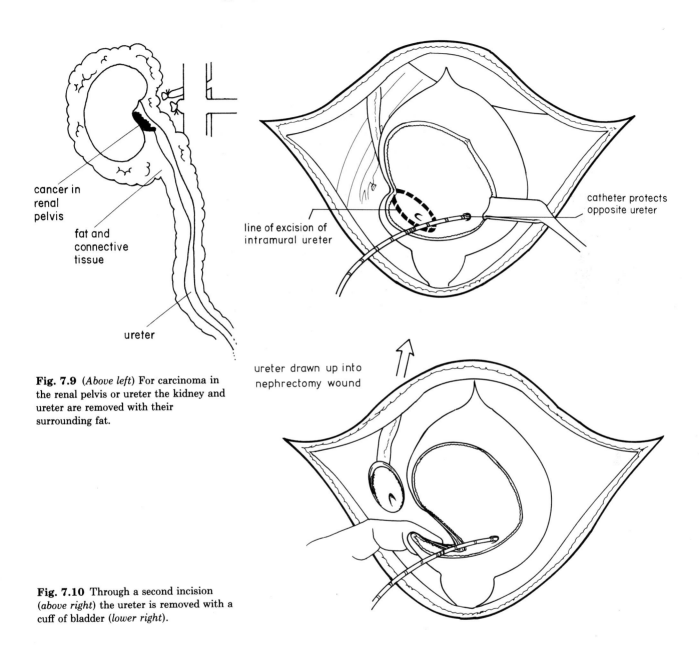

cancer in
renal
pelvis

fat and
connective
tissue

ureter

line of excision of
intramural ureter

catheter protects
opposite ureter

ureter drawn up into
nephrectomy wound

Fig. 7.9 (*Above left*) For carcinoma in
the renal pelvis or ureter the kidney and
ureter are removed with their
surrounding fat.

Fig. 7.10 Through a second incision
(*above right*) the ureter is removed with a
cuff of bladder (*lower right*).

ureter is then drawn up to the upper wound and both incisions are closed
with drainage.

Once cancer has appeared anywhere in the urothelium it may occur
again, so all these patients need regular follow-up with cystoscopy and
urography.

Nursing care

Although the nursing care is similar to that for radical nephrectomy, there are three main differences. The incision is unlikely to extend into the chest, so there is no need for an underwater sealed drain. Since a small part of the bladder around the intramural ureter is removed, a catheter is left in to drain the bladder for 8 to 10 days until the site is healed. A wound drain is left outside the bladder until drainage is negligible. It is wise to reinforce the doctor's advice about attending regularly for cystoscopy so that recurrences in the bladder may be detected and treated early.

Further reading

Blandy, J. P. (1986) *Operative Urology*, 2nd edn. Blackwell Scientific Publications.

Hendry W. F. & Bloom, H. J. G. (1985) Urothelial neoplasia. In *Textbook of Genito-Urinary Surgery*, vol. 1, eds Whitfield, H. N. & Hendry, W. F., pp. 971-1000. Churchill Livingstone, Edinburgh.

Woodhouse, C. R. J. (1987) Renal carcinoma. In *Scientific Basis of Urology*, ed. Mundy, A. R., pp. 311-326. Churchill Livingstone, Edinburgh.

8 Stone disease

Most calculi start off in the kidney but some of them work loose and get stuck in the ureter, or reach the bladder and then cannot get out.

Normal urine — after the glomerular filtrate has been processed in the tubule, ends up with an excessive amount of some solutes, notably calcium, oxalate, phosphate and urate which are all ready to precipitate in the urine as crystals, given half a chance. They will precipitate if there is any nucleus on which the crystals can grow — a dead papilla, another fragment of stone, or a foreign body such as a surgical suture. Like silt in a river, crystals tend to settle more easily if the urine is not flowing briskly — and so stones tend to form wherever there is obstruction or a stagnant pocket of urine and may be encouraged by prolonged bed rest.

The normal urine in most people in Britain is about 20 times supersaturated with respect to these salts and in summer and in hot climates, when there is excessive sweating, the urine becomes even more supersaturated, small wonder that stones are common. The real question is why do we not all make stones all the time, and the answer seems to lie in the presence of natural protective substances which keep the particles in suspension.

Metabolic causes of stones

In certain unusual conditions there is an even greater excess of solutes in the urine. The most important is the rare condition of *hyperparathyroidism* where overactivity of the parathyroid glands causes calcium salts to be taken from the bones into the blood stream, filtered into the urine, to be added to the existing excess of calcium in the urine. This is measured in a 24-hour collection made during a period of normal diet and activity (Fig. 8.1).

There are a number of other uncommon conditions in which an excessive amount of calcium finds its way into the urine (*hypercalciuria*) and some otherwise healthy people seem to absorb an excessive amount of calcium from their food and have hypercalciuria without any obvious cause for it — *idiopathic hypercalciuria.*

Another rare condition is *cystinuria.* Here a congenital abnormality prevents the renal tubules from reabsorbing a group of amino acids — cystine, ornithine, arginine, and lysine — from the glomerular filtrate. Of

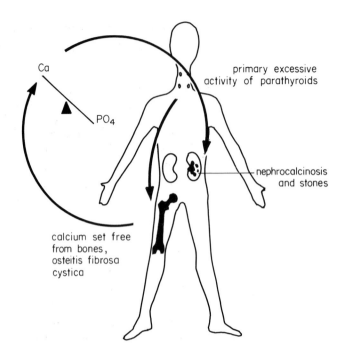

Fig. 8.1 When the parathyroid glands are overactive, calcium is taken from the bones into the bloodstream and filtered into the urine.

these, only cystine is insoluble, and forms stones in the urine which give a characteristic rather faint shadow on an X-ray because cystine contains sulphur. Cystinuria is an inherited condition. Stones may be prevented by giving penicillamine which joins to cystine to form a soluble by-product.

One interesting example of an excess of solute in the urine is seen in people who habitually make a very acid urine. Uric acid, one of the normal urinary solutes, is almost insoluble in an acid urine and precipitates out as a stone which is completely invisible to the X-ray. Uric acid stones can usually be prevented by taking alkalis (such as bicarbonate) to make the urine less acid, and drinking so much water that the urine never has a chance to become supersaturated but sometimes it is necessary to give allopurinol to prevent the formation of uric acid.

Infection and stone formation

Far more common than the metabolic stones are those which are caused by infection. Many microorganisms, and especially *Proteus mirabilis* convert urea into ammonia with the result that the urine becomes intensely alkaline. The phosphates which are normally present in urine are insoluble in an alkaline urine, and a mixture of magnesium and ammonium phosphate, usually mixed with calcium salts is formed. These stones are soft and crumbly and contain innumerable organisms. They can grow very rapidly and may come to form a complete cast of the renal pelvis and calices — a *staghorn calculus* (see below).

Presentation

The patient with a stone may present in several ways. The most dramatic is ureteric colic, when a small stone is making its way down the ureter. Sudden excruciating pain radiates from the loin to the groin, and is often followed by vomiting, sweating and abdominal distension.

When the stone is in the renal pelvis the pain is felt in the loin and may vary from mild discomfort to attacks of severe disabling pain, sometimes accompanied by haematuria.

Staghorn calculi may be surprisingly silent; they may only be discovered when repeated urinary infections are fully investigated. Usually the patient has felt tired and under par for some time, and infection and obstruction may have caused unsuspected and severe renal damage.

Stones in the bladder move about and scratch the sensitive trigone and patients experience pain referred to the tip of the penis or the vulva and a constant desire to pass urine, especially in the daytime.

Investigation of a patient with a stone

There are three steps:
1 To find out how many stones there are, where they are situated, and what damage they have done or are likely to do. Information is usually provided by an IVU, which will also show if there are any underlying reasons for stagnation of urine, e.g. outflow obstruction or a diverticulum in the bladder.
2 Metabolic causes of stones are ruled out, e.g. hyperparathyroidism, hypercalciuria, uric acid stone disease and cystinuria by measuring the quantity of these substances in the blood and in a 24-hour specimen of urine.
3 The urine is cultured to detect infection — particular attention being given to the presence of *Proteus mirabilis.*

Formation and growth of stones

Clumps of crystals collect in the tubules and gather under the tip of the papilla, until one day a crust of stone separates into the lumen of the collecting system, where it acts as the nucleus for further stone formation (Fig. 8.2).

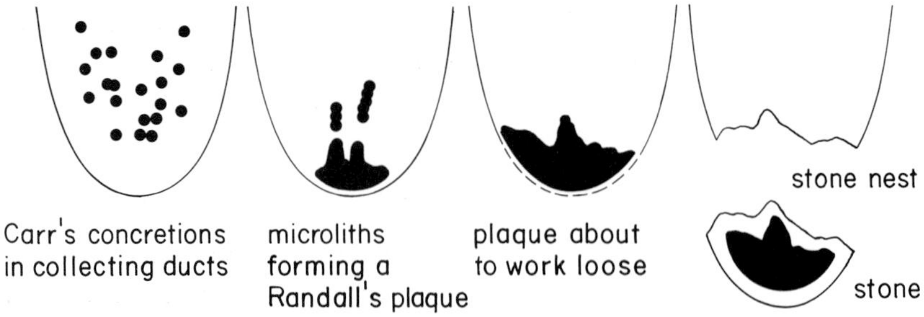

Fig. 8.2 Most stones begin in the papilla where the urine is most concentrated.

Carr's concretions in collecting ducts

microliths forming a Randall's plaque

plaque about to work loose

stone nest

stone

Once a stone has started to form in a renal calix it grows and progressively fills up the calix and later the pelvis until it forms a complete cast of the collecting system — a staghorn stone (Fig. 8.3).

Treatment of stones in the kidney

Tiny stones in an outlying calix seldom need any treatment at all. They may remain year after year without growing or giving rise to any trouble.

If they get loose and lodge in the renal pelvis or get so big that they cannot possibly go down the ureter, then they have to be removed.

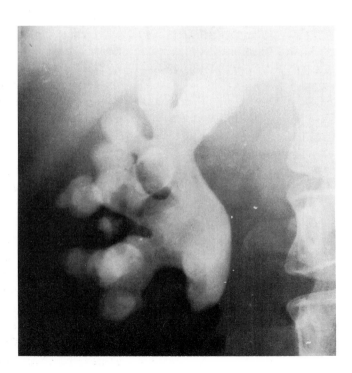

Fig. 8.3 A 'staghorn' calculus which has formed a complete cast of the renal pelvis and calices.

Nowadays there are three techniques for removing stones in the kidney — extracorporeal shock-wave lithotripsy (ESWL): the percutaneous technique (PCNL): and conventional open surgery.

Extracorporeal shock-wave lithotripsy — ESWL

This is the method of choice because it is relatively painless and free from many of the risks of any open surgical operation and needs far less time away from work — a few days instead of several weeks. There are several different types of ESWL machine now available.

The Dornier lithotriptor

This consists of a large bath containing an elliptical mirror with a powerful sparking plug at its first focus. The patient is anaesthetized and strapped into a chair which is lowered into the bath. A pair of X-ray machines allow the stone to be placed exactly at the second focus of the ellipse, and then a succession of sparks are let off which create powerful shock waves. Some of the shock is passed directly through the water to the skin and soft tissues, hence the need for anaesthesia. But part of the shock waves are reflected from the elliptical mirror and are concentrated at its second focus (Fig. 8.4) and break up the stone into smaller and smaller fragments which can then be passed down the ureter over a period of days or weeks.

If the urine is infected, a course of appropriate antibiotics is started on the day before treatment.

The shock waves sound like the report from a gun, so ear plugs are provided. The bladder is catheterized because a high fluid intake is maintained by intravenous infusion and it is necessary to prevent the patient from passing urine into the Dornier bathwater. The catheter is usually removed within 24 hours.

During the procedure an ECG is continuously recorded, as the shock waves are timed to coincide with the R (resistant) phase of the cardiac cycle; the leads are placed on the forehead and forearm, well out of the water. It is necessary to monitor the blood pressure carefully, as hypotension may occur due to the sitting position, the drugs that have been given and warmth.

Intravenous fluids are continued until the patient can take at least 2 litres orally without vomiting. As the pieces of stone are passed down the ureter there may be mild renal colic which can be relieved with diclofenac or co-proxamol. All urine is measured and filtered, and some fragments of stone kept for analysis. There may be some bruising at the site of exit of

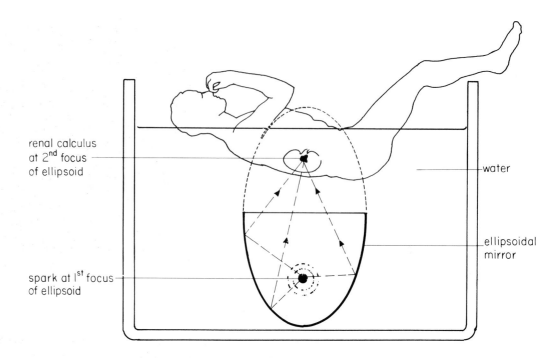

renal calculus
at 2nd focus
of ellipsoid

water

spark at Ist focus
of ellipsoid

ellipsoidal
mirror

Fig. 8.4 Dornier extracorporeal shock-wave lithotriptor: shock waves generated at the first focus are reflected off the ellipsoid mirror and meet at the second focus where the stone is lined up by means of two X-ray beams (not shown in the diagram).

the shock waves, but it seldom causes trouble and usually disappears within a few days.

The patient is usually up and about later on the day of treatment. The disintegration and passage of stones are monitored with ultrasound and plain abdominal X-rays.

COMPLICATIONS

The first treatment may not break the stone into fragments small enough to go down the ureter, and further treatments are often necessary. Each course of shock waves causes a certain amount of bruising in the loin, and the kidney may also suffer the consequences of haematoma — fibrosis and scarring. Very rarely cases have been reported where the kidney has been ruptured and haemorrhage has called for emergency nephrectomy. The main problem however is the presence of the fragments of stone blocking the lower end of the ureter — sometimes forming such a thick collection of sludge that it is necessary to pass a ureteroscope up the ureter to remove it (Fig 8.5).

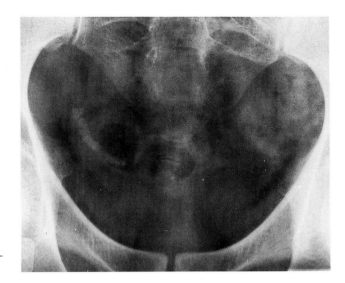

Fig. 8.5 The day after extracorporeal shock-wave lithotripsy: stone fragments are queuing up to pass out of the lower ureter — the 'steinstrasse'.

The Wolf 'Piezolith'

In this and similar second generation ESWL machines the patient lies on a spherical basin of water which is lined with many tiny piezoceramic devices from which the shock waves are focussed on the centre of the sphere (Fig. 8.6). Using ultrasound the patient is placed so that the stone lies at this centre. The shock waves do not hurt or bruise the skin, and

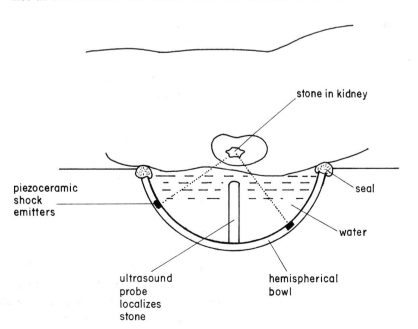

Fig. 8.6 Wolf 'Piezolith' extracorporeal shock-wave system. A spherical bowl is fitted with many tiny ceramic shock-emitters focused on the stone which is located by means of ultrasound.

they tend to crumble away the outer part of the stone instead of cracking it into larger fragments. This may require several sessions. The great advantage of this instrument is that it needs no anaesthetic, the patient does not need to be catheterized, and has no bruising or discomfort in the loin.

To make it easier for the fragments of stone to pass down the ureter a double-J stent (Fig. 8.7) is often passed into the ureter a day or two before the ESWL. This has the effect of making the ureter relaxed and wider. When the stones are very large, a tube may be placed into the kidney percutaneously before the patient is sent for ESWL.

Percutaneous nephrolithotomy — PCNL

Today this procedure may be employed in combination with ESWL. The patient is prepared for general anaesthesia and lies prone or on the unaffected side. Urethral and ureteric catheters are passed. Under X-ray or ultrasound control a fine guidewire is introduced into the kidney

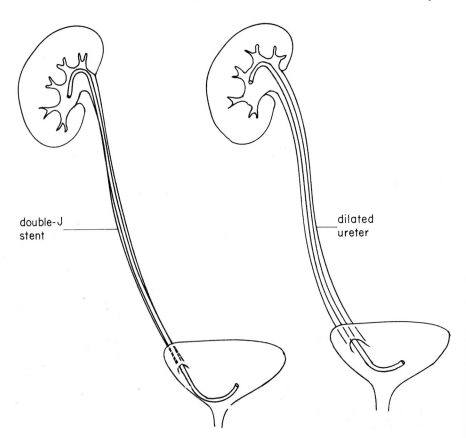

double-J stent

dilated ureter

Fig. 8.7 A double-J stent in the ureter causes dilatation which allows fragments of stone to escape.

through a lower calix, and over the guidewire a series of dilators (Fig. 8.8) are passed until in the end a 24 Ch sheath is introduced, through which small stones may be extracted with forceps. Larger ones are broken up by an electric spark with an *electrohydraulic lithotriptor* (Fig. 8.9), or a cylinder that oscillates at ultrasonic frequency to break up the stone — the *ultrasonic stone disintegrator* (Fig. 8.10).

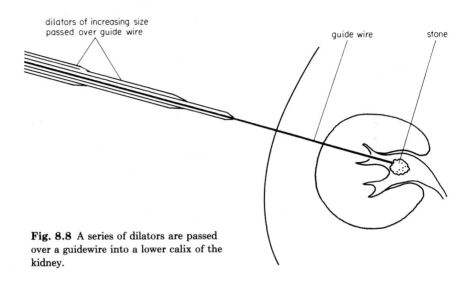

Fig. 8.8 A series of dilators are passed over a guidewire into a lower calix of the kidney.

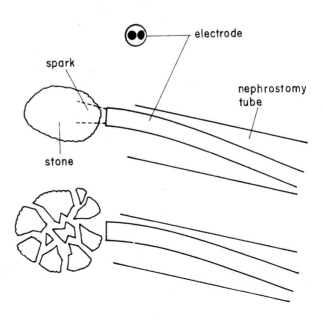

Fig. 8.9 Electrohydraulic lithotriptor: two electrodes emit a powerful spark which shatters the stone.

When the last tiny fragment of stone seems to have been removed a flexible *nephroscope* (Fig. 8.11) is introduced to make sure that no little bits have been left behind. A small nephrostomy tube is left in the kidney. The little incision does not even need a suture.

A day or two after the procedure a nephrostogram is performed by injecting contrast medium into the tube. Provided there is free drainage

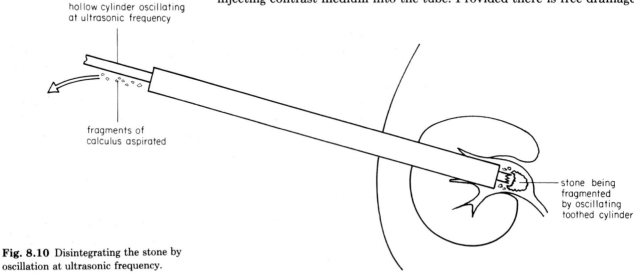

Fig. 8.10 Disintegrating the stone by oscillation at ultrasonic frequency.

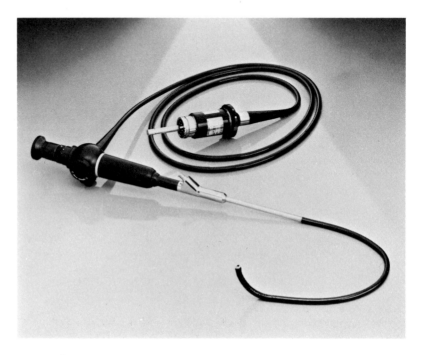

Fig. 8.11 A flexible nephroscope may be introduced through the nephrostomy tube to seek and remove residual tiny fragments of stone.

down the ureter, the tube is removed. Leakage settles down rapidly and the patient is able to go home.

PCNL can be complicated by haemorrhage, which is usually controlled by the insertion of the nephrostomy catheter. Infection and septicaemia can occur, as in any other urological procedure (see p. 48) and so appropriate antibiotic cover is used when the urine is known to be infected.

The patients spend a long time in one position on the X-ray table under anaesthesia, and are nursed in a similar position (on the unaffected side) afterwards, so that a sheepskin or sorbo ring should be provided to prevent a pressure sore.

Because the nephrostomy tube is smaller than the dilated track there is often a considerable leakage of blood-stained urine around it and the outer dressings need to be changed frequently in order to keep the patient comfortable and prevent infection.

Open removal of calculi

When these relatively uninvasive methods have failed or the stones are large and multiple they must be removed by conventional open surgery. If the incision goes through the renal pelvis the operation is called *pyelolithotomy*; if the kidney tissue has to be incised, it is called *nephrolithotomy* and in practice a combination of both is usually needed.

Under general anaesthesia, the kidney is approached through an incision along the bed of the 12th rib (Fig. 8.12). There is a bloodless space between the cortex and the renal pelvis which allows the cortex to be lifted

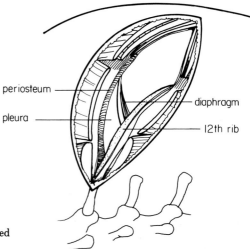

Fig. 8.12 The kidney is approached via the bed of the 12th rib.

off the renal pelvis so that it may be incised without bleeding or damage to the parenchyma (Fig. 8.13). The stones are removed completely, the calices thoroughly washed out and an X-ray is taken on the table in the operating theatre to check that no tiny fragments are left behind.

In a staghorn calculus when the stones are very large and fill the outlying calices with mushroom-shaped extensions it is necessary to incise the overlying cortex to get them out. To avoid accidentally cutting one of the segmental arteries they are localized with a Doppler ultrasound probe and the incision is made between them (Fig. 8.14) while a clamp on the renal artery cuts off the blood supply. The kidney is cooled to protect it from ischaemic damage with sterile ice slush, cooling coils or a trickle of ice-cold saline.

Nephrectomy

Even today stones are discovered so late that the kidney is virtually destroyed. Such a kidney is removed by the operation of *nephrectomy.*

Through the 12th rib-bed approach, the kidney is dissected from its surroundings (Fig. 8.15) taking care not to injure the colon and duodenum which lie immediately in front of it. The renal artery, vein and ureter are divided between ligatures and the mass is removed (Fig. 8.16).

Nursing care after pyelolithotomy, nephrolithotomy and nephrectomy.

The patient must be warned that it will be painful to cough or breathe deeply afterwards. This knowledge, combined with physiotherapy and the

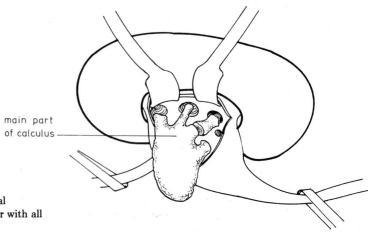

main part
of calculus —

Fig. 8.13 Through the bloodless plane between the renal parenchyma and the pelvis, the stone is removed together with all its outlying branches.

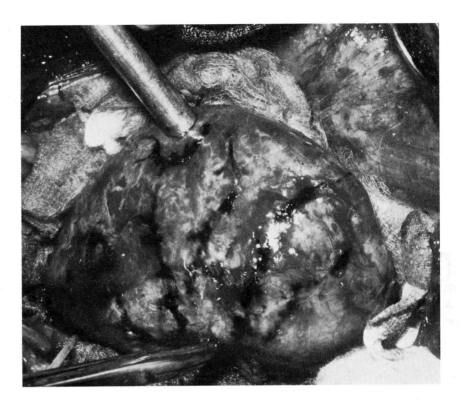

Fig. 8.14 A Doppler ultrasonic detector shows where the segmental branches of the renal artery are, so that outlying pieces of stone can be removed without bleeding.

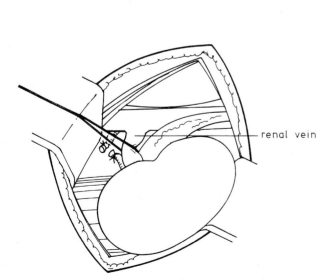

Fig. 8.15 When the function of the kidney is entirely destroyed by a stone it is removed; the renal artery is first divided.

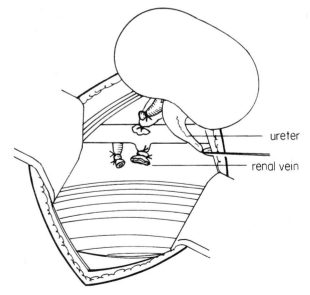

Fig. 8.16 Nephrectomy completed: the renal vein and ureter are divided.

assurance of regular postoperative analgesia, helps him to expand the lung bases fully and prevent postoperative *chest infection.*

A tube *drain* will be placed near the incision in the renal pelvis to remove escaping urine and serous fluid. It is attached to a drainage bag so that the fluid can be collected without the risk of infection or the discomfort of wet dressings, and it allows the amount to be recorded.

After an uncomplicated nephrectomy a drain is unnecessary. A kidney destroyed by stones is usually full of pus and difficult to dissect out, so a drain will be needed to avoid abscess formation.

After 4 or 5 days the drainage is minimal and a sleeve of fibrin has congealed around the track of the drain, which is now shortened and then removed. If a large volume of urine continues to drain it may be because a fragment of stone has become stuck in the ureter; an X-ray will confirm this and it may need to be removed endoscopically through the ureter.

Urethral catheters increase the risk of infection, and even though a little haematuria can be expected postoperatively there is seldom any need for a catheter. The day after operation the patient should be fit enough to get out of bed to pass urine or use the commode.

Intravenous fluids are given to maintain a urine output of about 2 litres during the day or two of reduced gut motility which results from irritation of the peritoneum after an operation on the kidney.

When the patient has passed flatus, one may give fluids and then whatever food the patient fancies.

There is also some risk of *haemorrhage* and blood transfusion may be required especially when it has been necessary to incise the parenchyma in nephrolithotomy.

A high *fluid intake* should be maintained indefinitely to reduce the stagnation and hyperconcentration of urine which may cause stones to form again. Patients should drink so much that they pass no less than 3 litres of urine per 24 hours. The type of fluid is immaterial — so long as it is mainly water. This is a very large volume and it needs effort and encouragement, and the need for it must be explained to them.

Patients find it interesting to see the stones that have been removed, and may want to show them off to family and friends. But they should not keep them as a trophy; every stone must go to the laboratory for analysis, and in the operating theatre a part is usually sent for microbiological culture.

The *stay in hospital* after an open operation on the kidney is about 10 days and 4 further weeks of convalescence are usually needed before returning to full activity.

When infected stones are present on both sides, the other side should be cleared as soon as possible so that the patient has a chance to be cured of the underlying infection with appropriate antibiotics to reduce the risk of recurrence.

Ureteric calculus

Most ureteric calculi are under 5 mm in diameter, and it has been shown repeatedly that stones as small as this have a better than 95% chance of passing down the ureter spontaneously, but as they do so, they give rise to pain — *ureteric colic*. This is caused in part by the dilatation of the ureter and pelvis upstream of the blockage, and partly by extravasation of urine into the surrounding tissues (Fig. 8.17). As a result of this extravasation there is often considerable abdominal distension and vomiting. When the pain is at its height patients should not be encouraged to drink, since this only makes the extravasation worse.

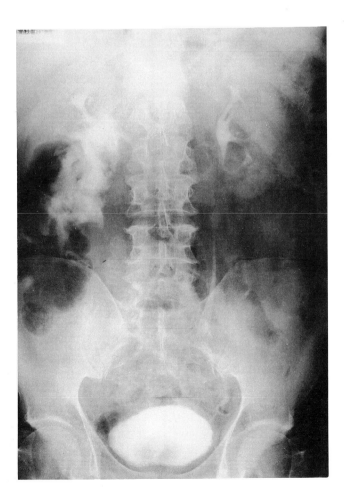

Fig. 8.17 A stone acutely blocking a ureter: urine containing the contrast medium has escaped into the surrounding tissues.

Patients with ureteric colic need urgent relief of their pain. Until recently it was necessary to prescribe large doses of morphine or pethidine, but recent experience shows that diclofenac (25 mg i.v. or 100 mg p.r.) gives even better relief without the risk of drug addiction.

Until recently most stones in the ureter were allowed to pass spontaneously and this is still the best treatment for many small stones but it may entail many episodes of colic. The process can be speeded up by pushing the stone back into the kidney by injecting saline up a ureteric catheter, passing a double-J stent (Fig. 8.18) and then destroying the stone as it lies in the renal pelvis by ESWL — the *push-bang* method. An alternative is to remove the stone endoscopically.

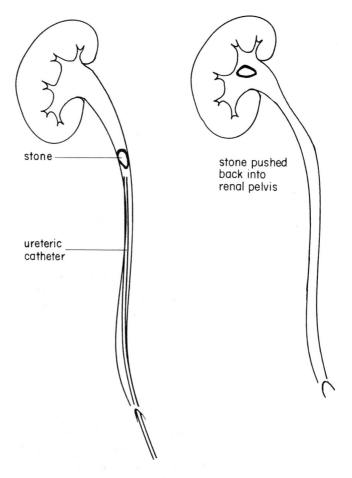

Fig. 8.18 Injecting saline up a ureteric catheter pushes a stone in the ureter back into the renal pelvis where it is treated by ESWL.

Endoscopic removal of ureteric stone

The Dormia basket

When the stone is near the lower end of the ureter, a catheter containing an ingenious basket (invented by the Italian surgeon Enrico Dormia) is passed via a cystoscope, up the ureter beyond the stone under X-ray control. When it has engaged the stone it is withdrawn (Fig. 8.19). This used to be a 'blind' procedure but today is more often performed through a ureteroscope.

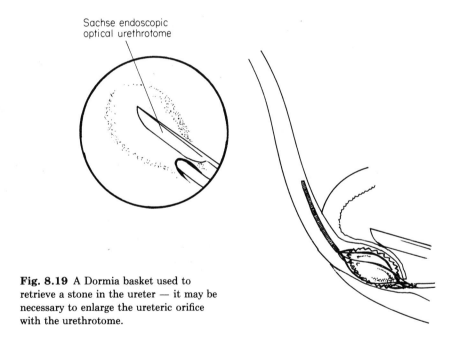

Sachse endoscopic optical urethrotome

Fig. 8.19 A Dormia basket used to retrieve a stone in the ureter — it may be necessary to enlarge the ureteric orifice with the urethrotome.

Ureteroscope

The ureteroscope — a long thin telescope — can be introduced up the ureter over a guidewire after first dilating it with bougies or a long inflatable balloon. The stone is seen through the ureterscope and caught in a Dormia basket. Larger ones are broken up with an electrohydraulic probe or an ultrasonic disintegrator (see p. 76). All procedures using the ureteroscope carry a risk of damaging the ureter, and if this occurs, a double-J stent is left indwelling for a few days to allow the hole to heal up.

Ureterolithotomy

It is still necessary to perform an open operation to remove some stones in the ureter when the stone remains stuck to the wall of the ureter. The procedure needs a general anaesthetic. Through the appropriate incision, the ureter is exposed, a sling is placed around the ureter upstream of the stone to prevent it slipping back into the kidney, the ureter is incised onto the stone and the stone removed. Usually the little incision in the ureter is left unsutured, a tube drain being placed down near the incision to let out the urine (Fig. 8.20). Drainage of urine may be considerable especially when there has been prolonged obstruction due to the condition of the ureter and post obstructive diuresis.

The drain is kept in for 5 days. After 5 days a track will have congealed around the drain and it can then be shortened, and removed a day or two later. Urine may escape from the drain site for a day or two but will then stop.

There is no difficulty collecting the urine immediately after the operation for the drain tube is led directly into a collecting bag. When the drain is shortened or has been removed, continued leakage of urine is managed by fixing an adhesive urostomy bag over the drain site. Note that the management of a urine drain is different to one which has been put in to let out pus, a drain is kept in so long as pus keeps coming out; drains for urine are left only so long as it is necessary for a track to form around them.

Stones in the bladder

Eventually most small stones work their way through the ureter into the bladder and are passed out through the urethra. If there is outflow

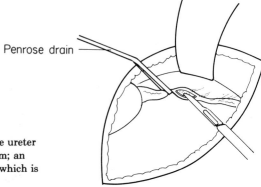

Fig. 8.20 Ureterolithotomy: the ureter is exposed behind the peritoneum; an incision is made onto the stone which is then removed.

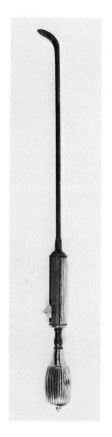

Fig. 8.21 The classical lithotrite.

obstruction (e.g. from enlargement of the prostate or a stricture in the urethra) then the stone cannot get out of the bladder but remains there and grows. Occasionally stones form in the bladder because of stagnation from outflow obstruction or on foreign bodies such as fragments of a catheter or a surgical suture.

These stones irritate the trigone and since its nerve supply is shared with that of the tip of the penis the pain is felt at the tip of the penis. After exercise the pain is worse and there may be haematuria.

Litholapaxy

Most bladder stones are removed endoscopically with a *lithotrite* (Fig. 8.21) an ancient instrument which crushes the stone into tiny fragments which are then washed out with an *Ellik evacuator* and cannula. There are more modern versions which allow the surgeon to see what he is doing, and through which the electrohydraulic or ultrasonic stone disintegrators can be passed (see p. 76). A catheter will usually be left in the bladder for a day or two, and the patient is encouraged to drink at least 3 litres of fluid.

Suprapubic lithotomy

It is most unusual for an open operation to be needed for a stone in the bladder except when modern equipment is not available or has been tried without success. The bladder is opened through a low abdominal incision and the stone is lifted out, the bladder is closed, and a urethral catheter is used for about 10 days while the bladder heals.

Further reading

Blandy, J. P. (1986) *Operative Urology*, 2nd edn. Blackwell Scientific Publications, Oxford.

Davidson, R. & McVey, P. (1985) Extracorporeal shock wave lithotripsy, *Nursing Times*, **Sept. 11**, 24–27.

Fitzpatrick, J. M., Murphy, D. M., Gorey, T., Alken, P. & Thuroff, J. (1984) Doppler localisation of intrarenal vessels: an experimental study. *British Journal of Urology*, **56**, 557–560.

Ford, T. F., Payne, S. R. & Wickham J. E. A. (1984) The impact of transurethral ureteroscopy on the management of ureteric calculi. *British Journal of Urology*, **56**, 602–603.

Marickar, Y. M. F. and Rose, G. A. (1985) Relationship of stone growth and urinary biochemistry in long-term follow-up of stone patients with idiopathic hypercalciuria. *British Journal of Urology*, **57**, 613–617.

Ryall, R. L., Darroch, J. N. & Marshall, V. R. (1984) The evaluation of risk factors in male stone-formers attending a general hospital out-patient clinic. *British Journal of Urology*, **56**, 116–121.

Segura, J. W., Patterson, D. E., LeRoy, A. J., May, G. R. & Smith, L. H. (1983) Percutaneous lithotripsy. *Journal of Urology*, **130**, 1051–1054.

Whitfield, H. N. & Mills, V. A. (1985) Percutaneous nephrolithotomy: a report of 150 cases. *British Journal of Urology*, **57**, 603–604.

Wickham, J. E. A., Miller, R. A. & Kellett, M. J. (1983) Percutaneous nephrolithotomy: results and cost effectiveness. *British Journal of Urology, Supplement*, 103–106.

Wickham, J. E. A., Webb, D. R., Payne, S. R., Kellett, M. J., Watkinson, G. and Whitfield, H. N. (1985) Extracorporeal shock-wave lithotripsy: the first 50 patients treated in Britain. *British Medical Journal*, **290**, 1188–1189.

9 *The kidney — diseases of the renal arteries and renal hypertension*

Aneurysm

There are three types of renal artery aneurysm (Fig. 9.1). The first two, the *fusiform* and *saccular* aneurysms may burst spontaneously and are operated on as soon as may be reasonably possible after they are diagnosed. The third kind — where there is an *arteriovenous malformation* — can pose certain difficulties; a small one may cause haematuria which may defy all methods of diagnosis. If it can be shown in an angiogram, the leak may be plugged with gelfoam but a partial nephrectomy may be needed. Larger arteriovenous fistulae may occur after stab wounds or a renal biopsy. The most common are those associated with a cancer of the kidney.

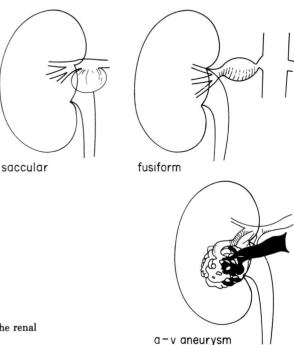

saccular   fusiform

a−v aneurysm

Fig. 9.1 Aneurysms of the renal artery.

Renal artery stenosis

Narrowing of the renal artery may give rise to an excessive release of renin from the kidney (see p. 12). The diagnosis is suspected in all young patients with hypertension. They often have an elevated level of renin in the blood and a narrowing in the renal artery is seen in the angiogram (Fig. 9.2). The blood pressure comes down if the action of angiotensin II is blocked by saralysin or captopril.

Transluminal angioplasty

A narrow balloon may be passed into the renal artery to dilate the narrow segment — *transluminal angioplasty* (Fig. 9.3). The preparation and nursing care are similar to those for a renal angiogram (see p. 27). The usual hypotensive therapy is usually omitted prior to treatment.

The procedure is not without its complications. The wall of the renal artery may split requiring an emergency operation to reconstruct the

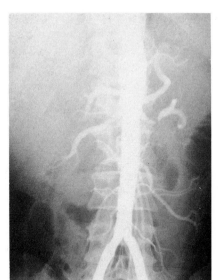

Fig. 9.2 Angiogram showing stenosis of the left renal artery.

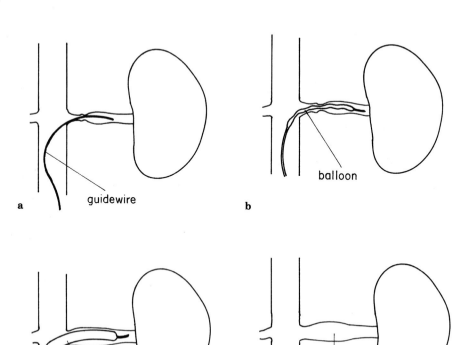

Fig. 9.3 Transluminal angioplasty: a balloon is manoeuvred over a guidewire into the renal artery and then expanded to enlarge the stenosis.

damaged vessel, and these possibilities are explained to the patient in the course of obtaining informed consent.

If transluminal angioplasty fails or seems inappropriate, the narrow part of the renal artery may be by-passed with a suitable graft (Fig. 9.4) or enlarged with a patch of vein (Fig. 9.5) but when the kidney is small and contracted it is best removed.

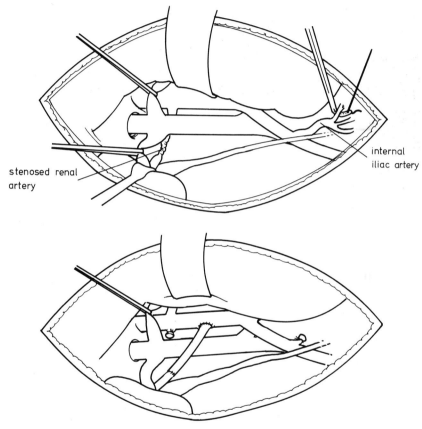

Fig. 9.4 For a stenosis of the right renal artery a graft has been taken from the internal iliac artery to by-pass the narrow segment.

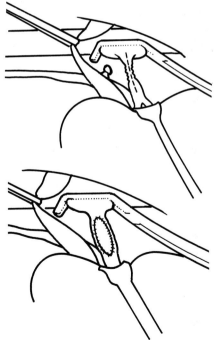

Fig. 9.5 The stenosed renal artery may be enlarged with a piece of vein.

Nursing care

Because the purpose of treatment is to lower the blood pressure, the main concern in the period after operations for renal artery stenosis may be a worrying phase of hypotension during which it may be difficult to know whether there is also haemorrhage. During this time it is important to be alert for a steadily rising pulse rate and any sign of bleeding from the wound, to measure the urinary output and make sure that at least 30 ml/h is produced. A catheter will probably have been left in the bladder for the first 24 to 48 hours. Intravenous fluids are needed in the postoperative period of paralytic ileus. Successful surgery results in a return to normal blood pressure levels without any medication.

Further reading

Blandy, J. P. (1986) *Operative Urology*, 2nd edn., pp. 73–74. Blackwell Scientific Publications, Oxford.

Buist, T. A. S. (1985) Percutaneous transluminal angioplasty in renal artery stenosis. In *Textbook of Genito-Urinary Surgery*, vol. 2, eds Whitfield, H. N. & Hendry, W. F., pp. 720–726. Churchill Livingstone, Edinburgh.

Snell, M. E. (1985) Surgical management of renal artery stenosis. In *Textbook of Genito-Urinary Surgery*, vol. 2, eds Whitfield, H. N. & Hendry, W. F., pp. 711–719. Churchill Livingstone, Edinburgh.

10 *Renal transplantation*

There are two steps in renal transplantation: (1) the removal of the *donor kidney*, and (2) grafting it into the recipient. The donor kidney may come from a living related donor or a cadaver.

Patients requiring renal transplantation will be nearing end-stage renal failure or already established on some form of dialysis treatment.

Donor nephrectomy from a living donor

These patients are under considerable emotional strain. They have been keyed up for many weeks, having once taken the decision to give a kidney to their brother, sister, son or daughter. They have undergone extensive investigations to make sure that they are free from infection and that both their kidneys are normal, and they will have had an angiogram to check that there is only one renal artery to the kidney selected for the transplant.

To get the kidney in the best possible state so that it works from the beginning in the recipient, the donor needs to be well hydrated and intravenous saline is started on the morning of the operation. Donors are warned that they may wake up with a small catheter in the bladder and that there will be pain in the chest, but that they will receive plenty of pain medication afterwards to enable them to breathe deeply and cough effectively. Although this will already have been discussed at length, patients like to be reassured yet again that they can manage with only one kidney and that the life expectancy of a patient with one kidney is just as good as with two.

The donor operation is carried out in one operating theatre while the recipient is made ready in a second. The kidney is approached through the 12th rib incision. A very careful dissection is made of the vessels going to and from the kidney. When the surgeon removing the donor kidney knows that the arteries and veins are satisfactory, the recipient operation is begun. When the recipient is ready, the donor renal artery and vein are ligated and cut and the donor kidney is plunged into ice-cold saline, irrigated with ice-cold preservative solution, and taken to the recipient theatre (Fig. 10.1).

The renal artery and vein are carefully checked in the donor, all bleeding is controlled, and the wound is carefully closed without a drain. If

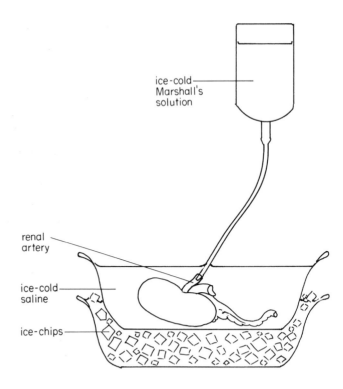

Fig. 10.1 When the donor kidney has been removed it is plunged into ice-cold saline and irrigated with ice-cold preservative solution.

the pleural cavity has been entered in the course of making the incision an underwater chest drain is left in for the first day or two.

Postoperative care

Donors all want to know as soon as possible whether the kidney they have given is working. This news is worth more than morphine to their morale and comfort. They will of course need pain medication during the first few days, but should be encouraged to be up and about to prevent deep vein thrombosis and pulmonary infection. Food and drink are given as soon as they have recovered from the immediate postoperative ileus — which lasts 24 to 36 hours. Visits to the recipient are mutually encouraging.

Removal of the kidney from a cadaver

Obtaining cadaver kidneys

Unless death is from sepsis, cancer, or kidney failure, those who care for the dying should always ask themselves — can the kidneys be used to save two lives? Doctors and nurses, especially those in accident and emergency departments, intensive care units and neurosurgical wards, should always be considering organ donation when it becomes evident that death is inevitable.

In the situation where the illness has allowed time for good relationships to be build up between relatives and staff, asking can be a natural progression of events. Increasingly, relatives broach the subject themselves and the wishes of the potential donors may be known. Even in an emergency, handled with sensitivity and honesty, the question can be asked. Relatives can be helped through their grief by the knowledge that their loss can be the gift of life for someone else.

Today there is no longer any question about the definition of death. A strict Code of Practice has been drawn up which makes it impossible for any person to be declared dead unless there is irreversible death of the brain. In *The Removal of Cadaveric Organs for Transplantation — a code of practice* (DHSS 1979, revised Feb. 1983) these rules are spelt out:

(i) The pupils are fixed in diameter and do not respond to sharp changes in the intensity of incident light.

(ii) There is no corneal reflex.

(iii) The vestibulo-ocular reflexes are absent.

(iv) No motor responses within the cranial nerve distribution can be elicited by adequate stimulation of any somatic area.

(v) There is no gag reflex or reflex response to bronchial stimulation by a suction catheter passed down the trachea.

(vi) No respiratory movements occur when the patient is disconnected from the mechanical ventilator long enough to ensure that the arterial carbon dioxide tension rises above the threshold for stimulation of respiration.

When death is determined on the basis of brain death, or where it is proposed to remove organs within an hour after respiration and circulation have ceased, death should be diagnosed by the following combination of doctors.

A consultant who is in charge of the case, or in the absence of a consultant, his deputy, who should have been registered for five years or more and who should have had adequate experience in the care of such cases, and one other doctor. Neither doctor should be a member of the transplant team, and the result of the examination and the diagnosis should be recorded in the case notes. The transplantation checklist attached to this code includes a model checklist of criteria for diagnosing brain death with space for two signatures.

It is customary to carry out the diagnostic tests on more than one occasion. As a patient must be presumed to be alive until it is clearly established that he is dead, the time of death should be recorded as the time when death was conclusively established, not some earlier time or a later time when artificial ventilation is withdrawn, or the heart beat ceases.

These careful rules ensure that the diagnosis of death is out of the hands of the transplant surgeon, and must be made by experienced doctors who are fully aware of the mistakes that can arise from previous administration of drugs, neuromuscular agents, hypothermia or metabolic conditions that might give rise to coma.

The *transplant coordinator* is called in as early as possible, and consideration is given to what organs other than the kidneys may also be used. Appropriate contact is made with other centres.

Once the medical decision has been taken, and the permission of the relatives has been obtained (and there are special rules laid down for those rare cases where it is impossible to contact them) every effort is made to preserve the kidneys in the best possible condition for donation. In this time of activity, the nurses have a dual role, to support and comfort the relatives, and to provide continued care for their patient, with discreet transfer to the operating theatre.

The relatives need the opportunity to say 'goodbye' as privately as practicable. Physical loneliness must not be allowed to add to their distress. Even though the person is dead and the death certificate has been issued, he or she may not look dead while still being ventilated. Further opportunity needs to be given even after the last offices have been performed to establish the reality.

The brain-dead donor should be kept well-hydrated and well oxygenated. Phenoxybenzamine may be given to prevent the vascular spasm which might impair the function of the kidneys, whilst of course having no ill-effect upon the donor.

This whole situation is inevitably traumatic for all the staff involved and as soon as possible the opportunity should be taken to relax and share feelings.

Cadaver donor nephrectomy

This is a difficult operation. To get good results it must be done carefully under optimum conditions. The brain-dead cadaver is taken to the operating theatre, and under conditions no less strictly aseptic than for any other open operation, the kidneys are removed through an abdominal incision (Fig. 10.2). Ventilation is kept up until the kidneys are removed so that they are not damaged by ischaemia.

The kidneys are perfused with ice-cold preservative solution which

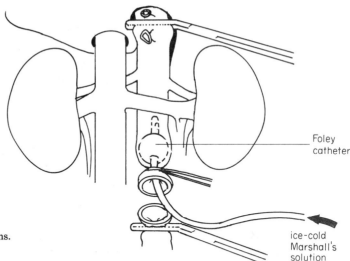

Foley
catheter

ice-cold
Marshall's
solution

Fig. 10.2 Removal of cadaver donor kidneys is a planned meticulous operation carried out with full aseptic precautions. The kidneys are irrigated with ice-cold solution to preserve their function.

has roughly the same composition as the fluid inside the cells of the body. After being perfused the kidneys are put into double sterile plastic bags, labelled, and packed in ice in which state they can be preserved and used for up to 36 hours — plenty of time for them to be transported to the hospital which has the best-matched recipient.

Kidney matching

We inherit from our parents one from each of their pairs of chromosomes. Chromosome pair number 6 (which is present in every cell of the body) is responsible for making the HLA antigens on the surface of every cell which, like number-plates on cars, can be recognized by the patrolling policemen of the body — the lymphocytes — when they are foreign to our bodies.

If the set of HLA antigens on the cells of the donor kidney is different from that of the recipient, the patrolling lymphocytes recognize the intruder, raise the alarm, summon assistance, and move in to kill the intruder. If the lymphocyte police succeed, the graft is *rejected.*

The action of the lymphocytes can be prevented by means of immunosuppressive drugs such as *azathioprine, cyclosporin A* and *prednisolone.*

When all the HLA antigens are matched correctly, many more transplants survive than when they are mismatched and so much effort is expended to try to match the donor to the recipient, even if this means delay and the transportation of kidneys over large distances. When a perfect match cannot be obtained immunosuppression permits prolonged survival of the graft, but the better the match, the better the likely outcome.

Putting in the donor kidney

Preparation of the recipient

When the good news is received that a kidney is available for a patient who has been waiting, often for many months, for a transplant, he is advised not to eat or drink, and come straight to the unit. It may be the midde of the night, he may be called from work or even from an exciting football match.

He will be excited, a little apprehensive, but full of hope of release from the restrictions imposed by dialysis or a poorly functioning kidney. He will probably be familiar with the unit and the staff, and know what to expect, but explanations are repeated and questions answered.

After a welcome and the sharing of initial feelings, blood is taken for a cross match to check that there are no cytotoxic antibodies to the donor kidney. (These are independent of the histocompatibility antigens which are already known, and the cross match usually takes about 2 hours).

During this time blood is taken for haemoglobin, WBC, urea and electrolytes as well as for blood transfusion cross matching and screening for titres of common viruses. An ECG and chest X-ray are also performed, as well as a general medical examination.

The nurse needs to admit her patient, and make preparation for emergency surgery speedily but thoroughly. Baseline cardiovascular observations are taken and recorded. It is important to identify any pre-existing infection, and swabs are taken from nose, throat, axillae and perineal areas. If the patient still has kidneys and passes urine a urine specimen is sent for microscopy and culture, and it is useful to note the volume of urine usually passed per day, so that it may be compared with the output after transplantation.

If overdue for dialysis, there may be time to haemodialyse the patient. In all cases, the presence of a *Cimino fistula* is clearly marked so that it can be protected and observed in theatre. If the patient is maintained on continuous ambulatory peritoneal dialysis (CAPD) the fluid is drained out, the line capped off and the dialysate sent for culture. The site of catheter insertion is inspected, swabbed and redressed. After all these procedures are completed the patient is weighed. If there is a tendency to constipation, 2 glycerine suppositories are given. The lower abdomen is shaved, and the patient is given a bath. After all this, the patient is grateful for premedication and a chance to relax before going to the operating theatre.

Anxious relatives may wish to stay at the hospital until the operation is safely over or will need to know when to telephone. A great deal may depend on the outcome for all the family.

The operation of transplantation

An incision is made in the iliac fossa of the recipient. The peritoneum is peeled back to expose the common and internal iliac artery and vein, and tapes are placed around them to cut off the blood during the operation (Fig. 10.3). Usually the renal artery of the donor kidney is joined to the internal iliac artery, but sometimes to the external iliac artery. The renal vein is anastomosed to the external iliac vein (Fig. 10.4). When the vascular anastomoses have been completed the immunosuppressive drugs are given intravenously, the tapes are undone, and blood is allowed to run through the kidney (Fig. 10.5).

All at once the cold, seemingly dead lump of kidney begins to expand and throb with life. The ureter begins to writhe and as urine oozes out of it, it is implanted into the bladder through a long oblique tunnel imitating the natural valvular entry of the ureter into the bladder that prevents reflux (Fig. 10.6).

The details of this procedure vary slightly from one hospital to another. Some leave a splinting catheter in the implanted ureter, some drain the wound and leave a catheter in the bladder.

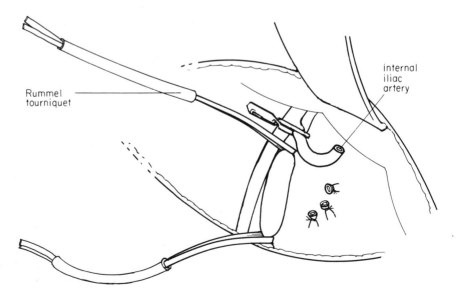

Rummel tourniquet

internal iliac artery

Fig 10.3 The renal artery may be anastomosed to the internal iliac artery.

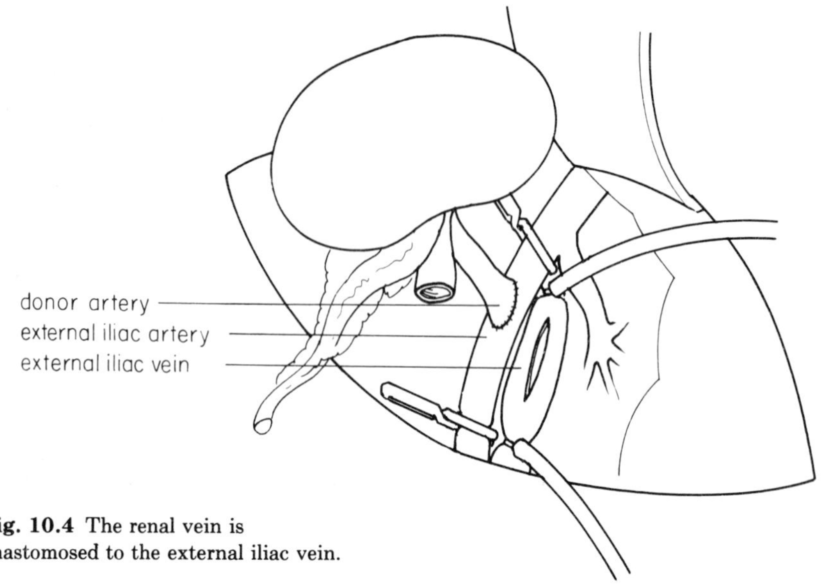

donor artery
external iliac artery
external iliac vein

Fig. 10.4 The renal vein is anastomosed to the external iliac vein.

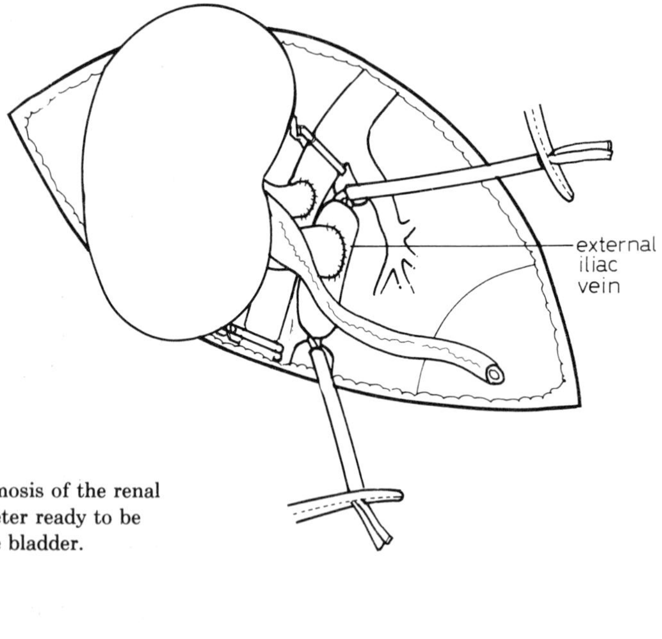

external iliac vein

Fig. 10.5 Anastomosis of the renal vein completed: ureter ready to be anastomosed to the bladder.

Immunosuppression

There are several regimes for immunosuppression. The standard scheme, developed over the last 25 years, uses a combination of *azathioprine* and *prednisolone*; the doses and timing vary from one unit to another, and are

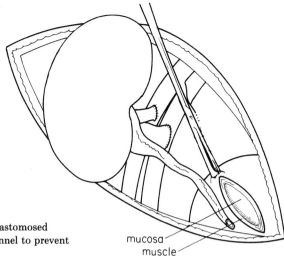

mucosa
muscle

Fig. 10.6 The ureter is anastomosed to the bladder through a tunnel to prevent reflux.

adjusted daily according to whether or not there is any evidence of rejection. In recent years *cyclosporin A* has been found to improve results at the expense of some impairment of renal function.

Normal progress after transplantation

Ideally the patient makes a speedy recovery from surgery, has little need of analgesia and produces normal volumes of urine with a good creatinine clearance. He is able to take what he likes to eat and drink from the first or second day, and soon develops a voracious appetite. There is no infection or rejection. He feels fitter and more mentally alert than he has for several years and may go home within two weeks, and is followed up in the clinic — at first every day — later on at longer intervals.

Not all patients are so fortunate, especially if they are diabetic or have complications such as severe atheroma. The risk of infection is increased by the use of immunosuppressive drugs. The nurse must be constantly on the look out for those small changes which may have great significance: pyrexia, glycosuria, breathlessness, diarrhoea, indigestion, cough or pain must all be reported, investigated and treated.

The patient must always be kept well informed of the reasons for investigations and changes in treatment so as to allay anxiety and encourage cooperation. After being responsible for their own treatment, rapid change and dependence, even with a positive and longed-for end in sight, can be quite frightening.

Postoperative care after renal transplantation

Immediate and early care

In the first few days close attention is paid to the risks of infection, haemorrhage, rejection and infarction, as well as to the careful monitoring of fluid balance and renal function. Immunosuppressive therapy is adjusted day by day.

Infection

Protective barrier nursing is often used after renal transplantation, and even if not, all staff, patients or visitors with colds or other infections, must be kept away from newly transplanted immunosuppressed patients. 'Opportunistic' infections are many and various.

Deep breathing exercises are encouraged and smoking is forbidden, to avoid chest complications. Sputum is immediately cultured, and any pyrexia promptly investigated.

Closed system drainage is used and this is never disconnected without good reason.

Haemorrhage and infarction

Major blood vessels are used for the anastomoses of the renal artery and vein. The suture lines may leak, and in acute rejection the kidney may swell so much that it actually splits. Any of these events will give rise to obvious bleeding, with pain, bruising and collapse of the patient. Blood transfusion and surgical exploration may be required.

Patients with renal failure often have atheromatous arteries, and indeed, endarterectomy may have been necessary at the time of the arterial anastomosis. It is necessary to check the pedal pulses and look out for any swelling of the legs especially on the side of operation. Anuria may indicate blockage of the renal artery or vein, which will infarct the transplanted kidney.

Fluids and renal function

At first, fluids are given intravenously, the type and volume depending on the patient's state of hydration, the serum level of potassium and the urine output. The output of urine is measured and recorded every hour until the volume is stable and thereafter less frequently, and it is all saved and sent to the laboratory every 24 hours for measurement of its urea, sodium, potassium and creatinine. Oral fluids may be given when they are tolerated.

PERSISTENT OLIGURIA

Some patients remain oliguric from *acute tubular necrosis*, and continue to need dialysis and a restricted diet and fluid intake for 2 to 3 weeks. In the absence of any other reason for concern, it is important to explain to the patient and the relatives that this is not unusual, and does not necessarily mean that the transplant will not be successful. During this period the patient must be kept as well as possible by dialysis. It is always encouraging to see some urine produced however small the volume.

DIURESIS

At the other extreme, some patients have an *excessive diuresis*, and lose large amounts of sodium and potassium. This is confusing for them; they see large volumes of fluid being given intravenously; they are asked to drink several litres a day, and to eat formerly 'forbidden fruits'. Careful explanation gains their cooperation and it always encourages them to see the 24-hour urine collection bottles fill up. During this time it is sometimes difficult for them to drink a lot, since the level of urea in the blood is falling, and the 'drive' that makes them thirsty is removed. These patients seem to be more at risk of rejection a week or so after the transplantation.

Management of the wound and the catheters

Units vary considerably in their use of catheters and drains. If a *ureteric splint* is used it is left for 10 days to maintain free drainage from the transplanted kidney and prevent the ureter from kinking while it heals. The *urethral catheter* is left for a further 2 days. These measures are thought to reduce the risk of leakage of urine but in many centres no ureteric splint is used and the urethral catheter removed much earlier. Specimens of urine from the catheters are sent for culture every day.

The *wound drain* usually remains for 5 or 6 days attached to a closed bag so that the fluid can be observed and measured. If there is more than a minimal leak of fluid or a reduced output of urine, one must suspect a leak of urine and as soon as there is any suspicion of this a specimen of the fluid is sent for measurement of its creatinine. If its creatinine is greater than that in the plasma the fluid must be urine.

The other fluid which may leak in large volumes from the transplant wound or drain is lymph. It usually looks rather darker than urine, is syrupy, froths on shaking and has the same creatinine content as the plasma. Although it is difficult to keep the wound dry and uninfected when there is a leakage of lymph, it is far less dangerous than a leak of urine — which usually calls for urgent reoperation. To keep the wound dry when there is a lymph leak a urostomy bag placed over the site will allow the fluid to be measured and avoid wet dressings.

Sutures remain for 2 weeks or longer since healing is often delayed in an anaemic and uraemic patient taking steroids.

Obstruction to the outflow of urine from the bladder should have been detected and corrected before transplantation, but it may only be diagnosed when the anastomosis starts to leak. The catheter is replaced, the fistula allowed to heal, and the outflow obstruction is put right at leisure.

Rejection

Immunosuppression

This varies from one unit to another. In most centres it starts with preoperative cyclosporin, and high doses of the azathioprine and prednisolone prior to release of the clamps at operation. Steroid doses are reduced gradually, and azathioprine and cyclosporin are carefully adjusted by reference to daily blood levels of cyclosporin, tests of renal function and blood count. They are prescribed daily.

In rejection, large doses of steroids are given intravenously.

Rejection may strike out of the blue at any time. The recipient's immunological police patrols of lymphocytes suddenly become aware of the foreign histocompatibility antigens on the cells of the donor kidney. They react by setting up 'road blocks' in the main vessels supplying the graft, sticking to the lining of the arteries of the donor kidney and forming a thrombus which slows the flow of blood until it finally ceases and the kidney dies.

Rejection may be acute and the patient very ill indeed, or it may be insidious and difficult to diagnose, especially when he is oliguric. Classically the patient is 'off colour' and not eating as well as formerly; there is a reduction in the output of urine, gain in weight, fever, raised blood pressure, tachycardia and tenderness over the graft. These signs are not all or always present and some patients feel surprisingly well. This is particularly true when cyclosporin A is used and a biopsy is needed when there is doubt.

In the early days after a transplant there are many other reasons why urine may not be formed and why the circulation through the kidney may cease: the anastomosis at the artery or the vein may block off, the operation site may become infected, or the implantation of the ureter into the bladder may become obstructed

Differential diagnosis

As soon as there is any doubt, investigations are called for; the kidney is scanned with DTPA and ultrasound, sometimes an angiogram is performed, fine-needle aspiration renal biopsy may be needed.

If the diagnosis of rejection is made, large doses of methyl prednisolone are given intravenously, and the dosage of cyclosporin checked remembering that it is itself nephrotoxic. At first these measures usually succeed in overcoming the reaction of the lymphocytes and the kidney recovers from their efforts to destroy it, but rejection may follow in episode after episode until, in the end it becomes irreversible, and the kidney dies because its blood supply has been completely blocked off. It should then be removed as soon as possible.

Nothing comes as such a blow to the patient whose hopes have been raised so high and who has already been through such an ordeal. But if the dead kidney is left in the pelvis, it is a perfect site for bacteria to grow in — and in a heavily immunosuppressed patient this can be very dangerous. Infection in the dead tissue may soften the site of anastomosis on the iliac artery and lead to catastrophic secondary haemorrhage.

In addition to prompt removal of the dead kidney, along with high doses of antibiotics, much understanding and encouraging support are given, as the patient returns to the life on dialysis from which he thought he had just escaped.

Second and third transplants

All is not lost if a transplant has failed. The patient can have second, third or fourth transplant. It is amazing how often people are willing to go through the experience of further transplantation in the hope of achieving a better quality of life than is possible with dialysis. Year by year the results show improvement; they will improve still further as more kidneys are provided from which to select more closely matched kidneys, and still better drugs emerge to combat rejection.

Further reading

Bishop, M. C. (1985) Renal transplantation. In *Textbook of Genito-Urinary Surgery*, vol. 2, eds Whitfield, H. N. & Hendry, W. F., pp. 1236–1257. Churchill Livingstone, Edinburgh.

DHSS (1979) *The Removal of Cadaveric Organs for Transplantation: A Code of Practice* (revised 1983). DHSS, HMSO.

Hamburger, J., Crosnier, J., Bach, J.-F. & Kreis, H. (1981) *Renal Transplantation: Theory and Practice*, 2nd edn. Williams & Wilkins, Baltimore.

Jennett, B., Gleave, J. & Wilson, P. (1981) Brain death in three neurosurgical units. *British Medical Journal*, **282**, 533–539.

Jennett, B. & Hessett, C. (1981) Brain death in Britain as reflected in renal donors. *British Medical Journal*, **283**, 359–362.

Morris, P. J. & Tilney, N. L. (Eds) (1984) *Progress in Transplantation*, vol. 1. Churchill Livingstone, Edinburgh.

Ward, E. (1984) Death or dialysis — a personal view. *British Medical Journal*, **289**, 1712–1713.

Weber, P. (1985) The human connection: the role of the nurse in organ donation. *Journal of Neurosurgical Nursing*, **17**, 112–119.

Wood, R. F. M. (1983) *Renal Transplantation — A Clinical Handbook*. Ballière Tindall, London.

11 *The ureter*

Anatomical relations

The ureter runs from the kidney to the bladder behind the peritoneum and the other viscera. It passes behind the vessels of the testis or ovary, in front of the common iliac artery and behind the superior vesical artery and, in the male, the vas deferens (Fig. 11.1).

Structure

The ureter is a continuation of the renal pelvis. It has the same waterproof transitional epithelium that lines the calices, pelvis and bladder, and is subject to the same kinds of urothelial cancer as the renal pelvis and

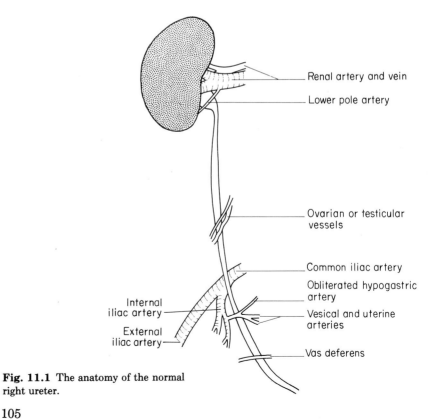

Fig. 11.1 The anatomy of the normal right ureter.

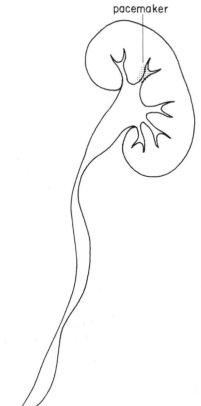

pacemaker

Fig. 11.2 The rate of ureteric peristalsis is governed by pacemakers in the renal calices.

urinary bladder. Its wall is made of smooth muscle fibres, each of which passes on its rhythmical contraction to its neighbour without the aid of nerves or ganglia.

The peristaltic contractions of the ureter pump urine down from the kidney to the bladder, to a rhythm set by a pacemaker in the renal calices according to the rate of formation of urine (Fig. 11.2). When there is obstruction downstream, the pelvis and ureter must work harder to pump the urine down to the bladder, so their muscles get bigger, coarser and stronger. Eventually the hypertrophied muscle becomes stretched and tired and so the ureter becomes dilated and its contractions ineffective. The ureter no longer can act as a pump, but merely as a drainpipe (Fig. 11.3).

Ureterovesical junction

The ureter runs obliquely through the wall of the bladder forming a valve to prevent urine in the bladder from running back up to the kidney (Fig. 11.4). This valve may be defective from birth or destroyed by disease and leads to recurrent urinary tract infection.

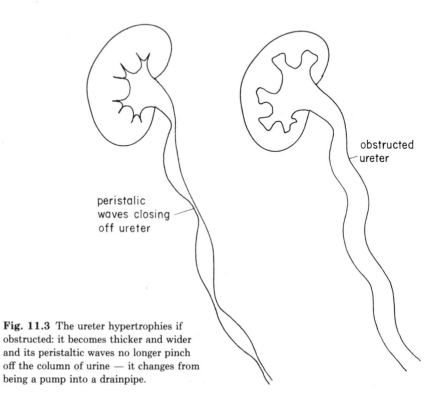

peristalic waves closing off ureter

obstructed ureter

Fig. 11.3 The ureter hypertrophies if obstructed: it becomes thicker and wider and its peristaltic waves no longer pinch off the column of urine — it changes from being a pump into a drainpipe.

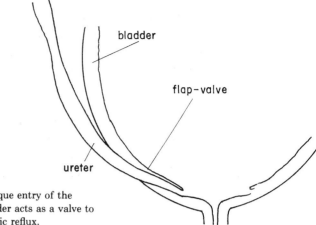

Fig. 11.4 The oblique entry of the ureter into the bladder acts as a valve to prevent vesicoureteric reflux.

The ureterovesical valve is tested by a *micturating cystogram*. The bladder is filled with contrast medium and the patient asked to pass water while the bladder is watched on an X-ray monitor. When the valve is diseased the urine may run up the ureter: minor degrees of reflux that involve only the lower ureter are of no importance but when they reach the renal pelvis and go right into the renal medulla — *intrarenal reflux* — then there is a risk of serious inflammation followed by scarring (see p. 45).

Blood supply

The ureter has a long thin artery running along its front which is supplied by a branch of the lower segmental artery of the kidney, and this is reinforced by branches from the lumbar arteries and the superior vesical artery (Fig. 11.5). The little vessel running along the ureter is thin and delicate; if it is stretched it gets thinner as does a rubber tube when it is pulled out. All operations on the ureter are planned to avoid tension.

Nerve supply

The nerves from the ureter convey sensations of pain. As they have a segmental pattern pain in the ureter from a stone is felt at progressively lower levels. Near the renal pelvis pain is felt in the distribution of T10 around the umbilicus. In the middle the pain is felt in the distribution of L2 and 3 — the groin or knee — and in the lower third the sacral dermatomes make the patient want to urinate and feel pain in the vulva and tip of the penis (Fig. 11.6).

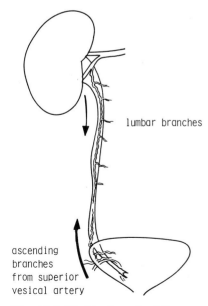

Fig. 11.5 The blood supply of the ureter.

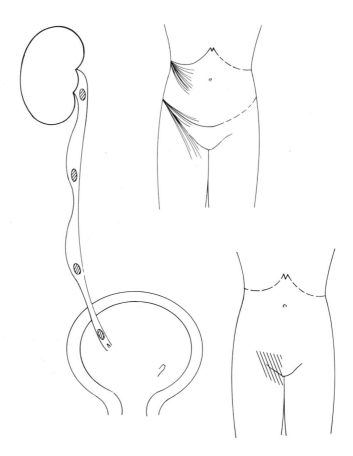

Fig. 11.6 Pain from a stone is felt at different levels, as it makes its way down the ureter.

Another curious feature of pain involving the ureter is the disturbance of intestinal function that occurs; obstruction or infection of the ureter can give rise to severe abdominal distension and vomiting.

Diseases of the ureter

Congenital anomalies of the ureter and duplex

A group of abnormalities of the ureter may appear as a result of early branching of the ureteric bud in fetal life (see p. 38). With a duplex ureter the ureter from the upper half-kidney may open downstream of the sphincter causing incontinence of urine, or it may enter the bladder in a little balloon — a utererocele — which can cause obstruction. The ureter from the lower half-kidney may open into the bladder through such a short tunnel that it cannot act as an efficient valve, and allows urine to run up to the kidney — *vesicoureteric reflux* — with pain, repeated urinary infections and consequent renal damage. These ureters are reimplanted in such a way as to prevent reflux (see p. 48).

Pelviureteric junction obstruction and hydronephrosis

Although sometimes seen in infants, this condition is usually detected in adult life. There is a stiff ring of scar tissue just where the renal pelvis narrows down to form the ureter — *pelviureteric junction (PUJ)* (Fig. 11.7). Nobody knows why this ring of scar tissue forms just there. When only a small volume of urine is being made by the kidney, the lumen of the pelviureteric junction is big enough to allow the urine to run down the ureter, but if the patient drinks a large amount of fluid and so has a diuresis, it is not large enough, and urine begins to accumulate under pressure upstream of the narrow segment: the renal pelvis is stretched and the patient experiences colicky pain in the loin, often with vomiting. This is often mistakenly diagnosed as indigestion and it is surprising how many investigations for their pain these patients have often undergone with negative results.

The diagnosis is made by the IVU (Fig. 11.8). If in doubt, a diuretic such as frusemide is given to attempt to wash out the contrast in the distended pelvis. The same information can be obtained with the renogram

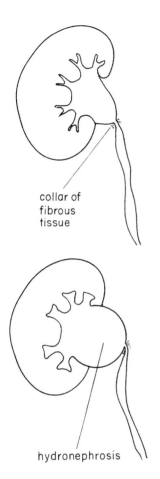

collar of fibrous tissue

hydronephrosis

Fig. 11.7 In idiopathic pelviureteric obstruction a rigid collar of fibrous tissue around the ureter allows only a restricted flow of urine; in diuresis the renal pelvis becomes distended.

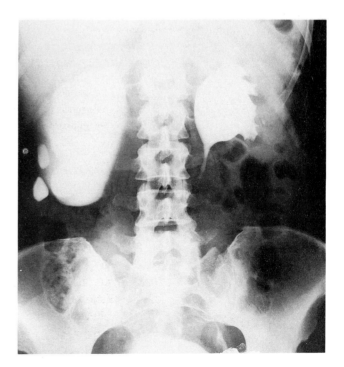

Fig. 11.8 Excretion urogram showing typical appearance of bilateral hydronephrosis from pelviureteric junction obstruction.

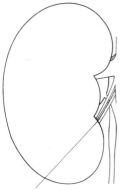

lower polar
segmental artery
and vein

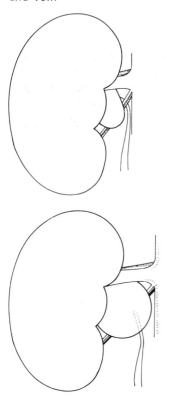

Fig. 11.9 The distended renal pelvis
may bulge out in front of the lower pole
vessel.

(see p. 35) combined with frusemide, and in exceptional cases if there is still doubt, Whitaker's test is used (see p. 35). If the diagnosis is confirmed, *pyeloplasty* is performed.

Pyeloplasty

This is generally performed on young and otherwise fit patients who recover well. The kidney is approached either through a 12th rib-bed incision or an anterior incision made so as to avoid the peritoneum. The renal pelvis is seen to be distended and often bulging forwards between the branches of the renal arteries giving the misleading impression that the inferior segmental artery is causing the obstruction (Fig. 11.9). There are several versions of this operation, but all have the same aim — to let a long U-shaped gusset of the surplus renal pelvis into the narrow top of the ureter so as to widen it (Fig. 11.10). A splinting catheter such as a *Cummings tube* may be left across the anastomosis to prevent kinking. This is allowed to drain freely for 8 or 9 days and is then clamped. Provided there is no pain, pyrexia or leakage in the next 24 hours, the tube is removed. A little leakage from the site is then to be expected. In general the nursing care is as for pyelolithotomy (see p. 78).

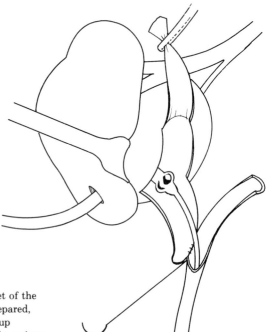

Fig. 11.10 Pyeloplasty: a gusset of the surplus renal pelvis has been prepared, which will be sewn into the slit-up upper end of the ureter over a Cummings tube that serves as a splint as well as a safety valve.

If there is pain or a fever when the tube is clamped, the clamp is removed. There may be a brisk flow of urine which causes the patient to jump. If so, a nephrostogram is performed — contrast medium is injected into the Cummings tube while its passage is monitored on an X-ray screen to make sure there is neither obstruction nor leakage.

Trauma to the ureter

Although *penetrating* and *closed injuries* of the ureter are described, and any missile or knife wound can damage the ureter, these are rare lesions, which are found and repaired by the surgeon exploring the penetrating wound or the closed abdominal injury. They may heal up too tightly and give rise to a ureteric stricture.

Iatrogenic injury

This is the most common form of ureteric injury seen in hospital today. It may follow hysterectomy, caesarian section, or some other operation in the pelvis where the ureter is accidentally crushed in a forceps, caught up in a stitch, or tied in mistake for an artery (Fig. 11.11). In the last few years the ureteroscope has added to the list of causes of ureteric injury.

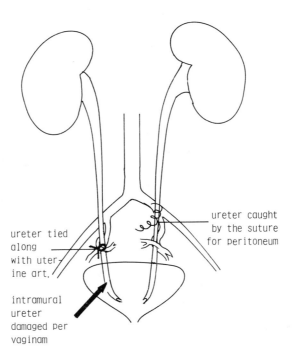

ureter caught by the suture for peritoneum

ureter tied along with uterine art.

intramural ureter damaged per vaginam

Fig. 11.11 Accidental operative injury to the ureter.

Diagnosis

If the injury has not only damaged but obstructed the ureter the patient will have pain in the loin. If the urine is infected, there will be high temperature as well as pain. The diagnosis should be confirmed at once by an emergency IVU.

More often, the injury is not noticed for 4 to 5 days, until the tissues that have been crushed or ligated undergo necrosis and give way, and urine leaks through the upper end of the vagina. The first person to realize that something has gone wrong is usually the patient, who finds fluid oozing from the vagina. The nurse must acknowledge that something may be wrong and that it will be investigated and put right.

The first step is to make sure that the suspicious fluid is urine. A small amount of it is collected, and the laboratory asked to measure its creatinine. Urine is the only fluid in the body that can possibly have a creatinine greater than that of the blood, so this simple test establishes beyond doubt that the fluid is urine.

The next step is to discover where the leak is, and close it. In former days it was customary to distinguish between leaks in the ureter and the bladder because the former were repaired early, the latter after a delay of 6 to 8 weeks. It is now clear that delay is undesirable in either condition, and the patient is returned to theatre as soon as she is reasonably well.

These youngish patients are understandably never happy about going through a second operation made necessary as a result of the first. Delay does not improve matters and they easily become demoralized by a prolonged period of distressing incontinence. They should be referred to a urologist as soon as it is confirmed that the leakage is of urine. Reassure them that the leak can be put right.

An IVU is performed at once; it usually shows some dilatation of the side where the ureter is injured. Next, under general anaesthesia cystoscopy is performed to make sure that there is not also a hole between the bladder and vagina — a *vesicovaginal fistula* (see p. 158). A bulb-ended catheter is placed first in one ureter, and then in the other, and contrast medium injected under X-ray control (Fig. 11.12) to show whether either or both ureters have been damaged.

Repair of ureterovaginal fistula

The abdomen is then reopened through the previous incision and the injured ureter traced down to the site of the damage where it is freed from surrounding adhesions (Fig. 11.13). A U-shaped *Boari flap* is made from the wall of the bladder. This is designed long enough to bridge the gap

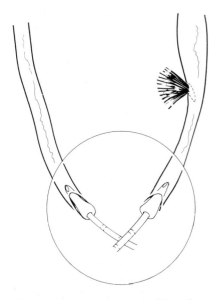

Fig. 11.12 A ureterogram is obtained on each side with a bulb-ended catheter.

without any tension. The ureter is led through a tunnel under the mucosa to prevent reflux and sutured over a splinting catheter (Fig. 11.14). The flap is sewn up and the wound closed with a drain to the outside of the bladder and a catheter inside it.

The drain is removed in 48 hours, the splinting catheter and sutures after 10 days, and the urethral catheter a day or two later. Note that the ureteric splinting catheter is led out of the abdomen on the side opposite

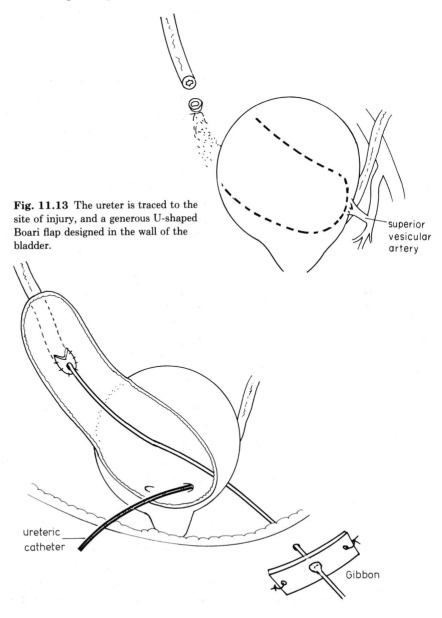

Fig. 11.13 The ureter is traced to the site of injury, and a generous U-shaped Boari flap designed in the wall of the bladder.

superior vesicular artery

ureteric catheter

Gibbon

Fig. 11.14 The ureter is joined to the Boari flap with a tunnel to prevent reflux over a splint.

the ureter which has been reimplanted to prevent it from kinking. If this splint becomes obstructed, the patient will have pain in the loin on the operated side. After repair of a vesicovaginal fistula (see p. 158) ureteric catheters may be placed on both sides, and it is important to be aware they cross over.

After a second pelvic operation there is an increased risk of deep venous thrombosis and pulmonary embolism. Elastic stockings, subcutaneous heparin, leg exercises and early mobilization help to prevent this calamity.

Three months later the bladder will have completely remodelled itself so that the site of the reimplantation into the Boari flap is almost impossible to detect.

If a *vesicovaginal fistula* is found, this also is repaired there and then (see p. 158).

Inflammations

Although the urothelial lining of the ureter is probably involved in most cases of acute pyelitis it always heals without scarring. Only in *tuberculosis* (see p. 162) and in *bilharziasis* (see p. 162) does the inflammatory process damage the wall of the ureter to cause narrowing in tuberculosis and either dilatation or narrowing in bilharziasis.

Idiopathic retroperitoneal fibrosis

This very curious condition has no known cause (though there are many theories). A stiff white patch of scar tissue forms behind the peritoneum, obliterating the aorta and vena cava, compressing and drawing the ureters in towards the midline (Fig. 11.15). Patients have backache, hypertension, vague general illness and a raised sedimentation rate. The diagnosis is so unspecific that it is often some time before anyone thinks of asking for an IVU.

Some patients present with rapidly deteriorating renal function if both ureters are involved. On these occasions the obstruction is temporarily relieved by percutaneous nephrostomies on each side (see p. 74) which give time for the patient to recover and be made ready for surgery. This benign kind of fibrosis must be distinguished from similar fibrosis set up by cancer in the retroperitoneal tissues.

To make the diagnosis usually requires laparotomy. At this operation the ureters are freed from their tight surrounding corset of fibrous tissue and wrapped up in soft omentum, which allows them to writhe about and pump urine again, as well as preventing the return of the fibrous tissue

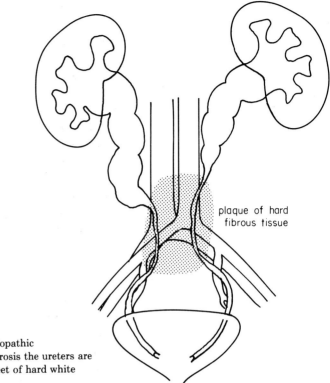

plaque of hard
fibrous tissue

Fig. 11.15 In idiopathic
retroperitoneal fibrosis the ureters are
caught up in a sheet of hard white
fibrous tissue.

(Fig. 11.16). The operation invariably leads to a period of ileus. Relief of
the obstruction may result in a diuresis so that in the early days after
operation the maintenance of fluid and electrolyte balance is important.
Thereafter a quick and usually full recovery is expected.

The fibrous tissue may resolve with hydrocortisone so if the diagnosis
is certain steroids may be given so long as a close look-out is kept for their
side-effects. Steroids are sometimes used in combination with surgery.

Cancer of the ureter

Primary carcinoma of the ureter

The ureter, being lined with urothelium is apt to form urothelial cancers
which, like those of the renal pelvis and bladder are of three grades of malignancy. In the good grade G1 it is possible to be conservative and remove
only the tumour while saving the kidney and ureter. In the bad G3
tumours, the entire kidney and ureter must be removed, probably
combined with preoperative radiotherapy as well, because the lining of the

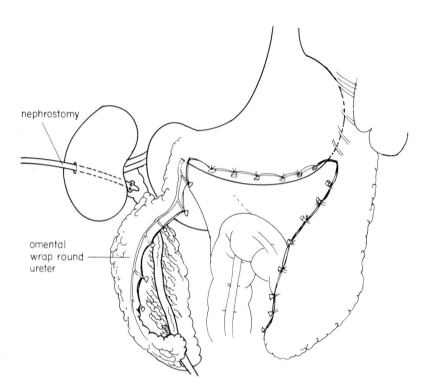

Fig. 11.16 After the ureter has been freed from the fibrous tissue it is wrapped up in omentum to prevent recurrence.

ureter is so thin that the tumour has often invaded the retroperitoneal tissues by the time the diagnosis is made so that the outlook is bad. The nursing care is as for carcinoma of the renal pelvis (see p. 66).

Secondary cancer involving the ureter

The ureter is frequently invaded by cancer arising in the prostate gland. This (see p. 214) is often amenable to hormone treatment and it is worthwhile to carry out a temporary decompression with a *double-J* splint of silicone rubber. This is introduced under general anaesthesia through a cystoscope over a guidewire (Fig. 11.17) which is pushed up into the renal pelvis and checked by X-ray to be in the correct position. These double-J tubes can be left in position for up to 3 months without becoming obstructed and they are easily removed or replaced through a cystoscope depending on response to treatment.

Percutaneous nephrostomy

A very similar object can be achieved if a guidewire is introduced via a needle under local anaesthesia into the distended renal pelvis. Once the

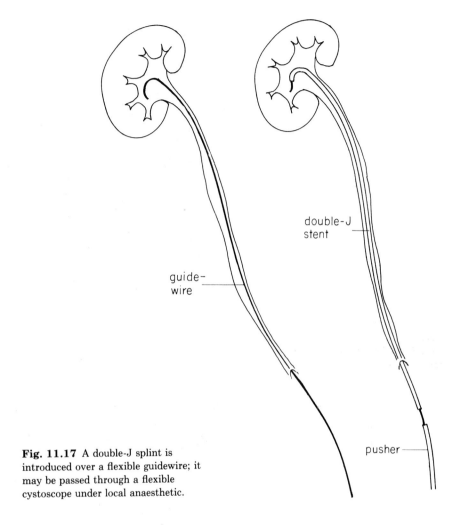

Fig. 11.17 A double-J splint is introduced over a flexible guidewire; it may be passed through a flexible cystoscope under local anaesthetic.

guidewire is in position, a silicone rubber tube is passed over it into the kidney (Fig. 11.18), and may be left in position for months — long enough for the cancer of the prostate to respond to treatment. This is obviosuly more difficult for the patient who may need help in managing the drainage bag, and may find the nephrostomies rather uncomfortable.

When other cancers such as carcinoma of the cervix or rectum invade and obstruct the ureters there is little that can be done to cure them. The team looking after the patient must be careful not to meddle; a patient who would otherwise die a painless death in uraemic coma may be snatched back from a peaceful sleep only to die in prolonged discomfort a few weeks later.

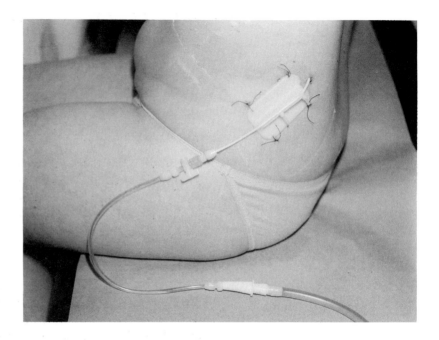

Fig. 11.8 Percutaneous nephrostomy in place. Note 'plate' used to maintain position and prevent kinking of tube.

Ureteric calculus

Having described these different forms of obstruction to the ureter, it is wise to remember that the most common cause of obstruction to the ureter is a calculus — and that most of the more rare and exotic ureteric conditions can be mimicked by a stone — especially one that is not opaque to X-rays (see p. 67).

Further reading

Blandy, J. P. (1986) *Operative Urology*, 2nd edn. Blackwell Scientific Publications, Oxford.

Blandy, J. P. & Tiptaft, R. C. (1985) Benign and malignant retroperitoneal fibrosis. In *Textbook of Genito-Urinary Surgery*, vol. 1, eds Whitfield, H. N. & Hendry, W. F., pp. 319–328. Churchill Livingstone, Edinburgh.

Bowsher, W. G., Shah, P. J. R., Costello, A. J., Tiptaft, R. C., Paris, A. M. I. & Blandy, J. P. (1982) A critical appraisal of the Boari flap. *British Journal of Urology*, **54**, 682–685.

Flynn, J. T., Tiptaft, R. C., Woodhouse, C. R. F., Paris, A. M. I. & Blandy, J. P. (1979) The early and aggressive repair of iatrogenic ureteric injuries. *British Journal of Urology*, **51**, 454–457.

Gosling, J. A. & Dixon, J. S. (1985) Embryology of the urinary tract. In *Textbook of Genito-Urinary Surgery*, vol. 1, eds Whitfield, H. N. & Hendry, W. F., pp. 123–131. Churchill Livingstone, Edinburgh.

Whitaker, R. H. (1985) Megaureter. In *Textbook of Genito-Urinary Surgery*, vol. 1, eds Whitfield, H. N. & Hendry, W. F., pp. 309–318. Churchill Livingstone, Edinburgh.

12 *The bladder — structure and function*

Structure

The bladder is a hollow organ which lies in the pelvis behind the pubic symphysis, in front of the vagina, uterus and rectum. It has two parts — an expansile vault and a fixed, triangular base — the *trigone* (Latin = triangle). The ureters enter at two corners of the *trigone* and the internal opening of the urethra lies at the third — the *internal urinary meatus* (Fig. 12.1).

When distended, the bladder rises into the belly, and can be felt on abdominal palpation. As part of the collecting system it is made of the same material — i.e. smooth muscle lined with a waterproof urothelium. The muscle of the wall of the bladder is called the *detrusor* (Latin = pusher-out). The urine is pushed out through the urethra, which is different in the two sexes.

Female urethra

The female urethra is about 5 cm long, surrounded by two rings of muscle, an upper involuntary ring made of smooth muscle — the *bladder neck*, and a lower voluntary one made of the striated muscle of the pelvic floor. They work together as the *sphincter mechanism* of the bladder (Fig. 12.2).

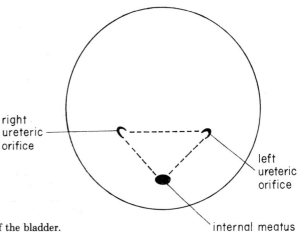

right
ureteric
orifice

left
ureteric
orifice

internal meatus

Fig. 12.1 The trigone of the bladder.

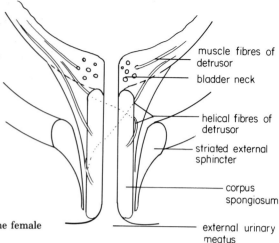

Fig. 12.2 The structure of the female urethra.

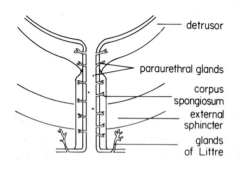

Fig. 12.3 Many tiny paraurethral glands open into the female urethra.

The upper part of the female urethra is lined by the same urothelium as the bladder, while the lower part is lined by squamous epithelium like that of the vagina, so that it is equally affected by changes in oestrogen activity with age and the menstrual cycle. Many tiny 'paraurethral' glands empty into the urethra (Fig. 12.3).

Male urethra

In males the urethra is longer and more complicated because between the upper and lower sphincters it is surrounded by the *prostate gland* (see p. 197) which is made up of many little secreting glands which open into the urethra (Fig. 12.4).

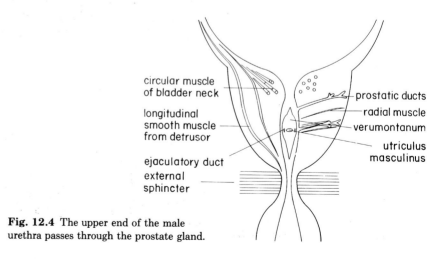

Fig. 12.4 The upper end of the male urethra passes through the prostate gland.

At the lower end of the prostate gland the urethra becomes very thin (the *membranous urethra*) where it passes through the lower striated voluntary sphincter to enter the *corpus spongiosum* which now surrounds it to the tip of the *glans penis* where the urethra opens on the *external urinary meatus*, hooded by the foreskin or *prepuce* (Fig. 12.5).

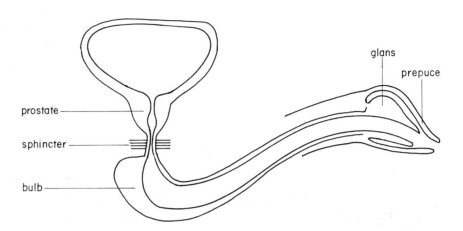

Fig. 12.5 Anatomy of the male urethra.

Function

The purpose of the bladder is to hold a reasonable quantity of urine, and then expell it all at a convenient time. Normally, when one wants to urinate the *detrusor muscle* contracts at the same time as both the sphincters relax (Fig. 12.6).

When the bladder is full, stretch receptors in the detrusor muscle send signals up the pelvic parasympathetic nerves to the *spinal centre for the bladder* in the second and third sacral segments of the spinal cord. They are found at the level of the first lumbar vertebra.

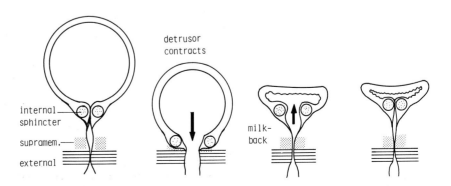

Fig. 12.6 Normally as the detrusor muscle contracts so the sphincters relax.

When the message that the bladder is full reaches the S2 and S3 segments in the spinal centre there are two results:

1 Impulses go down the pelvic parasympathetic nerves to make the detrusor muscle contract to empty the bladder.

2 The normal continual flow of nerve impulses along the parasympathetics to the upper, internal sphincter and along the pudendal nerve to the lower, voluntary sphincter is cut off.

This coordinated activity in the S2 and S3 segments of the cord is modified by higher centres in the brain via pathways in the spinal cord. We all know that when we are bursting to pass water but it is inconvenient to do so — we can suppress the process by conscious effort — *central inhibition*. We also know that under emotions such as anxiety or terror there may be an urgent need to empty the bladder — *central facilitation*.

Unfortunately the control centre for this complicated system is situated in a very vulnerable position, just where the rigid thoracic spine joins the flexible lumbar spine which is where the back is most apt to be injured in traffic or industrial accidents (Fig. 12.7).

If this S2/S3 control centre is destroyed by a piece of broken bone its reflexes are wiped out. The detrusor and the sphincters are paralysed, and

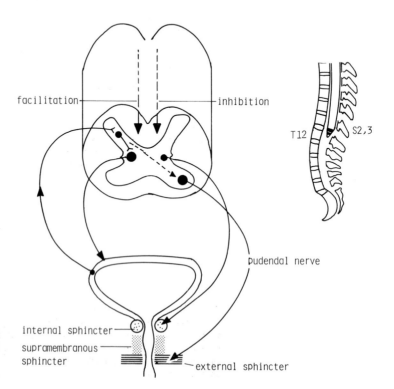

Fig. 12.7 The spinal centre for the bladder is in S2/S3 at the tip of the spinal cord, at the level of the T12 vertebral body.

the bladder is converted into a floppy bag which constantly leaks but never quite empties out, and inevitably becomes infected (Fig. 12.8).

Much the same happens if all the nerve fibres connecting the bladder and sphincters to the spinal cord are injured by operations in the pelvis or diabetic neuropathy — the spinal centre can receive no message from the distended bladder, nor send orders to the detrusor and the bladder becomes huge and atonic (Fig. 12.9).

The pathways between the S2 and S3 segments and the brain may be damaged or irritated in multiple sclerosis, spinal tumours, disk lesions or spinal injury. On one hand the conscious brain may not be able to inhibit

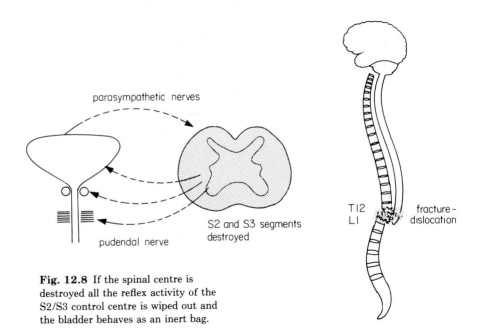

Fig. 12.8 If the spinal centre is destroyed all the reflex activity of the S2/S3 control centre is wiped out and the bladder behaves as an inert bag.

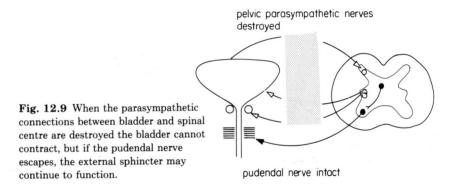

Fig. 12.9 When the parasympathetic connections between bladder and spinal centre are destroyed the bladder cannot contract, but if the pudendal nerve escapes, the external sphincter may continue to function.

the micturition reflex, and on the other a lesion that irritates these connecting tracts in the cord, may set off the reflex (Fig. 12.10).

In practice there are many variations on these basic disorders of the nervous control of the bladder.

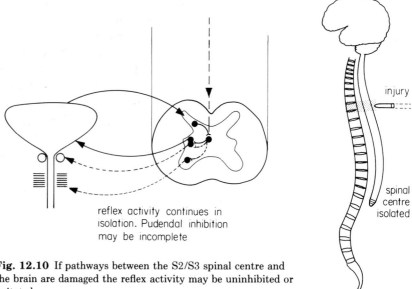

reflex activity continues in isolation. Pudendal inhibition may be incomplete

injury

spinal centre isolated

Fig. 12.10 If pathways between the S2/S3 spinal centre and the brain are damaged the reflex activity may be uninhibited or irritated.

Investigation of the bladder

Cystoscopy

Rigid cystoscopy

The cystoscope is the classical instrument of the urologist. It is essentially a long thin telescope, illuminated from a powerful light source conducted by a flexible bundle of glass fibres, each fibre coated with glass of a different refractive index so that all the light shone in one end bounces its way along the inner glass fibre and emerges at the other end (Fig. 12.11)

Different telescopes provide different views of the inside of the bladder, and a wide range of accessories make it possible to take a biopsy, pass a catheter into a ureter, remove small tumours and crush stones in the bladder. Cystoscopy may be performed under local anaesthesia but if anything further has to be done general anaesthesia is needed. It is not necessary to shave the perineal area.

Flexible cystoscopy

If one winds coated glass fibres on a wheel, glues them, and cuts them across (Fig. 12.12) the two cut ends will have the same arrangement of glass fibres, so that not only light, but an image made up of thousands of little dots like a TV screen may be transmitted down the flexible bundle of fibres. This is the principle of flexible endoscopes used today in the oesophagus, stomach, bronchus, biliary tree and colon and most recently of all — the bladder. Flexible cystoscopy is painless. It is performed in outpatients under local anaesthetic. Its most important role is in the follow-up of patients with bladder cancer. The procedure is much like catheterization, with minimal discomfort from the feeling of fullness from the irrigant solution (Fig. 12.13).

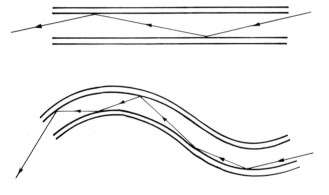

Fig. 12.11 In a flexible fibre-light cable each thin glass fibre is coated with glass of a different refractive index; all the light entering one end emerges at the other.

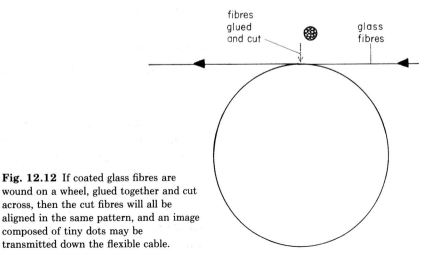

fibres
glued
and cut

glass
fibres

Fig. 12.12 If coated glass fibres are wound on a wheel, glued together and cut across, then the cut fibres will all be aligned in the same pattern, and an image composed of tiny dots may be transmitted down the flexible cable.

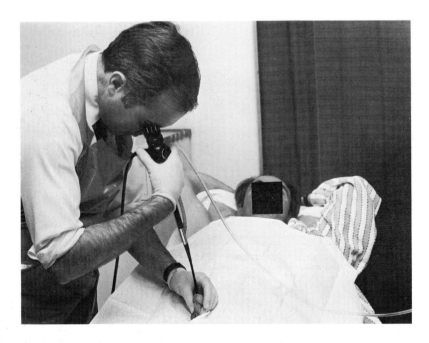

Fig. 12.13 Flexible cystoscopy is painlessly performed under local anaesthesia (courtesy of Mr C. G. Fowler).

Cystogram

Contrast medium in the bladder gives a useful picture of its shape. For most purposes enough reaches the bladder in an ordinary IVU to show if the detrusor muscle has become thick and sacculated as a result of hypertrophy, and measure how much urine is left behind after the patient has tried to pass water — *residual urine*. Much the same information can be obtained by ultrasound. To reveal the details of a diverticulum the contrast medium is injected through a fine catheter (Fig. 12.14)

Cystometrogram

After the patient has voided, two fine tubes are passed into the bladder. One is connected to a manometer that measures pressure, the other leads to a bottle of dilute contrast medium which is run in steadily and allows a radiographic picture of the patient passing water to be recorded at the same time as the pressure inside the bladder. Sometimes it is necessary to subtract the pressure inside the abdomen (from a fine tube placed in the rectum) to give the *subtracted pressure* due to the detrusor (Fig. 12.15). Often these measurements are combined with a cystogram — the *videocystourethrogram* or *VCU* which records the appearance and the pressures in the bladder at rest and during micturition (Fig. 12.16).

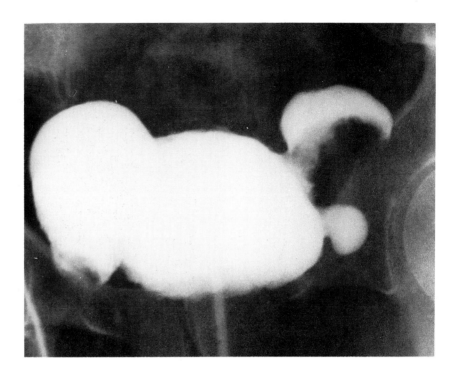

Fig. 12.14 Contrast medium injected into the bladder gives a shadow of the bladder — in this case showing a tumour in a diverticulum.

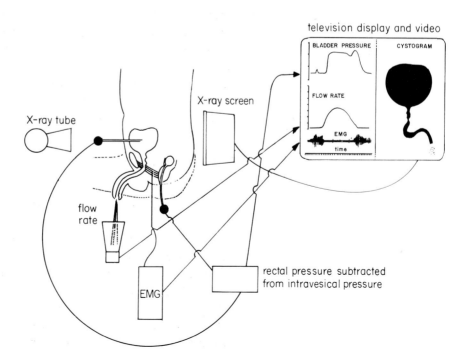

Fig. 12.15 Videocystometrography.

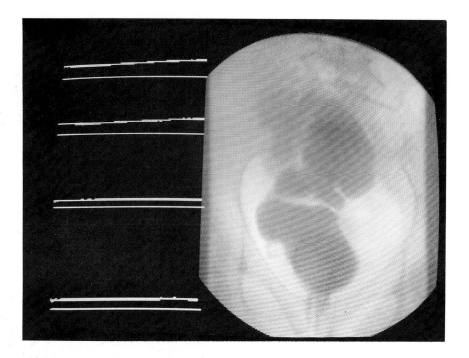

Fig. 12.16 The pressure in the bladder and the flow rate is recorded on the same TV screen as the cystogram.

Sphincter electromyography — EMG

When it is suspected that the pelvic floor is not being relaxed in coordination with the contraction of the detrusor, fine needle electrodes are inserted into the muscle through the perineum, which give a continuous record of their electrical activity (Fig. 12.17). The electrodes are exceedingly fine and their insertion almost painless, but the thought of having any needles placed anywhere is always worrying.

Patients are embarrassed as it is by their incontinence, and may be even more troubled by the prospect of undergoing urodynamic investigations which may be routine for the staff in the urology department but bizarre and even terrifying for the patient. A confident, individualistic approach, careful and patient explanation, and an opportunity to ask questions are essential.

Personal clothing could get wet and should be exchanged for a hospital gown. Privacy and modesty must be respected as far as possible and the fewer people present the better. Catheterization for both men and women may be slightly uncomfortable, as is the sensation of fullness when the bladder is filled with volume that is a little more than usual, and the presence of needle electrodes in the perineum. When the bladder is full, the catheters are removed.

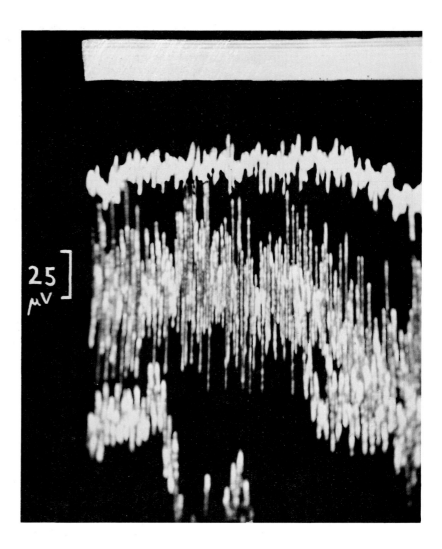

Fig. 12.17 Sphincter electromyogram: the 'spikes' record the electrical activity of muscle fibres.

Men are asked to stand up and void into a flow meter; when there is obstruction to the outflow from the bladder, the urine comes out more slowly than normal. The *flow rate* is recorded by a flowmeter and recorded on the same record as the VCU (Fig. 12.18).

Women who suffer from stress incontinence have X-ray screening lying and standing and are asked to cough while their bladder is full. A vaginal examination may also be needed, and there is often some embarrassing leakage of urine. It is very reassuring for them to know that this is entirely to be expected and that the urodynamic team are all used to these problems and the cause of their incontinence will be clearly demonstrated.

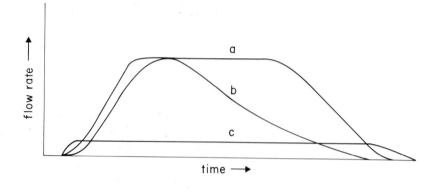

Fig. 12.18 Urine flow rates recorded on a 'uroflowmeter': (a) normal, (b) prostatic hypertrophy, and (c) urethral stricture.

Fig. 12.19 The pressure in the urethra is recorded as the catheter is slowly withdrawn, giving a measure of the pressure in different parts of the urethra — the 'urethral pressure profile'.

Nerve conduction studies

Sometimes the trouble lies in the nerves connecting the bladder to the spinal cord. To measure the speed a nervous impulse passes along these connections a stimulator may be placed in the bladder or vagina and sensitive detectors over the spinal cord or in the brain itself to record the *bladder evoked responses*. In some diseases the speed of transmission of these messages is slowed down. This test can be quite painful and patients need to be warned what to expect.

Urethral pressure profile

The pressure along the urethra may be measured if a catheter connected to a pressure recorder is slowly withdrawn. It measures the increase in pressure at the internal and external sphincter — the *urethral pressure profile* (Fig. 12.19).

Further reading

Gosling, J. A. & Dixon, J. S. (1985) Upper urinary tract: structure. In *Textbook of Genito-Urinary Surgery*, vol., 1, eds Whitfield, H. N. & Hendry, W. F., pp. 279–285. Churchill Livingstone, Edinburgh.

Turner-Warwick, R. T. & Whiteside, C. G. (1979) Clinical urodynamics. *Surgical Clinics of North America*, **6**, 1–304.

13 *Incontinence*

Urinary incontinence may be defined as the involuntary leakage of urine in inappropriate places at inappropriate times which becomes a social and hygienic disability.

Incontinence is very common and occurs in varying degrees, but whatever the degree, it causes much distress, embarrassment, inconvenience, hard work and expense, and at worst it can be socially crippling. At last it is receiving greater attention and is being discussed more openly. Manufacturers are responding to the need for more efficient appliances and the appointment of Incontinence Nursing Advisors is at least an acknowledgement that more needs to be done in education and the coordination of patient care.

The urological team has a very important role to play in its assessment, its correction (where possible) and the alleviation of difficulties when no cure is possible. At the end of the day there will still be some patients for whom there is no urological treatment or operation. For them it may be necessary to alter a pattern of behaviour or life-style or change the emphasis on the attention that they receive.

The patient needs to have equipment he or she can manage, as well as support in terms of adequate supplies and laundry that will allow him or her to cope with confidence. Quite simple practical matters such as the ability to undo clothes quickly enough, the degree of mobility, and whether or not there is a toilet and washbasin within easy reach at home, all need to be considered in the management of incontinence.

There are three types of urinary incontinence:

1 Where there is an abnormal opening for the urine, e.g. an ectopic ureter or an abnormal *fistula*.

2 Where there is an error in the nervous function of the bladder.

3 Where there is a mechanical defect in one or both the sphincters.

In order to differentiate between these a careful history is necessary, noting the age of the patient, the onset, severity and pattern of symptoms and the general physical and mental state of the patient, including emotional stress. The side-effects of any drugs that are being taken may well be relevant, as is any tendency to constipation. Incontinence may be underplayed or exaggerated, so that observation and recording the pattern of incontinence is important.

For many patients just to listen and to acknowledge that they have a problem can bring tremendous relief and may be the first step on the road to continence and new found confidence.

Analysis and culture of the urine may reveal unsuspected diabetes or infection, either of which may aggravate incontinence. An IVU (p. 21) and urodynamic investigations (p. 126) are often needed to make a diagnosis.

Abnormal opening for the urine

Ectopic ureter

In a duplex system (p. 38) the ureter from the upper half-kidney may enter the urethra downstream of the sphincter apparatus. The children are wet day and night. Curiously, the wetness is often unnoticed until puberty.

Fistulae

Fistulae may occur after gynaecological operations when a hole is made between the ureter and the vagina (p. 111), or between the bladder and the vagina (p. 158), and they may occur after neglected obstructed labour.

Other fistulae follow operations on the urinary tract when urine continues to leak from a drainage track or from the wound but they persist only if there is obstruction downstream of the organ from which the urine is issuing — e.g. a stone stuck in the ureter down from an incision in its wall, a foreign body such as a nylon suture in the track of the fistula or cancer or tuberculosis or previous radiotherapy that prevents the track from healing up (Fig. 13.1).

Fistulae may be investigated by injecting contrast medium into the opening with a syringe and fine catheter — *fistulogram* (Fig. 13.2). They can be managed temporarily with urostomy appliances.

The treatment of a fistula is directed to correcting the underlying cause: obstruction must be relieved, a foreign body removed, and cancer or tuberculosis must be treated appropriately. Very occasionally it is necessary to excise and close off a fistula because its tract has become lined with epithelium from one end to the other. This is rarely seen except in association with strictures of the urethra.

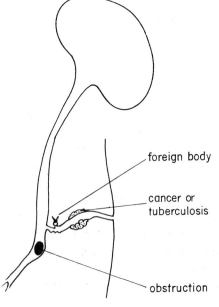

foreign body

cancer or tuberculosis

obstruction

Fig. 13.1 (*Left*) Urinary fistulae close of their own accord unless there is an obstruction downstream, or some other disease such as cancer, tuberculosis or a foreign body that prevents healing.

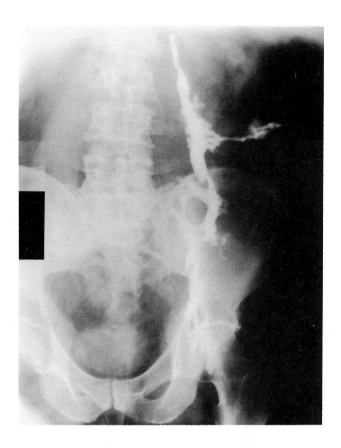

Fig. 13.2 To show the track of a fistula, contrast medium is injected into one or more of its external openings to obtain a fistulogram.

Errors in the nervous control of the bladder

Errors in education and training

Bedwetting

Anyone who has ever had to train a puppy will know that a baby animal empties the bladder whenever it is full. This is the simple uncomplicated reflex working. With encouragement and training, the puppy learns first to inhibit this reflex in the daytime and wait until he is taken outside, later he learns to inhibit it at night.

The same sequence occurs in children; first they learn to inhibit the reflex by day, later on at night — but this depends on part of the brain keeping awake while the rest is sleeping. This is more difficult for some perfectly healthy children than for others, and it is not abnormal to wet the bed occasionally even at the age of 9 or 10.

Anything which tends to increase the stimulus coming up from the stretch receptors in the bladder, e.g. when the urothelium is inflamed because of infection — will make it more difficult to inhibit, therefore infection must be ruled out.

Treatment of bedwetting aims to do three things:

1 To reinforce the normal daytime inhibition over urination. The child is encouraged to pass water when he wants to rather than when his bladder seems full, to exercise and reinforce the inhibition circuits.

2 To establish a conditioned reflex. A simple electrical device consisting of two tinfoil plates separated by the undersheet of the child's bed is connected to a battery and a buzzer (Fig. 13.3). If the sheet is soaked with urine the buzzer goes off and the child should be woken up and put on his pot. In this way the inhibition of the reflex is reinforced, and the child learns to associate the messages from his full bladder with the need to wake up and pass water. Parents and child must be fully informed and co-operative, and the parents must play their part and really make sure that the child wakes up. Praise reinforces success.

3 The child may be given medication to lighten the level of sleep. The trouble is that children quickly get used to the tablets, requiring larger and larger doses. Medication works best in conjunction with the two other techniques.

Oversensitive reflex arc

When the bladder is filling there may be an unwanted and unexpected contraction of the detrusor long before the bladder is full. One reason for

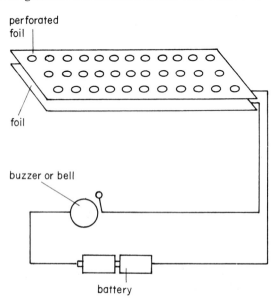

Fig. 13.3 The 'bedwetter's buzzer': an alarm bell is sounded when urine makes contact between the foil plates which are placed between the sheets under the child.

this may be that the afferent limb of the reflex arc is getting an unusually strong signal from the bladder because there is an inflammation or a stone, and no matter how hard the patient tries, the reflex arc cannot be inhibited (Fig. 13.4). This is known as 'urge incontinence' and in the presence of an indwelling catheter — 'bladder spasm' (see p. 210).

Another reason is that the reflex arc may be too sensitive because it is being *facilitated* from centres higher up in the spinal cord or brain, (Fig. 13.5) or because the normal nervous pathways down which the inhibitory signals come have been interrupted (Fig. 13.6). A cystometrogram (p. 126) will show that the detrusor is contracting long before the bladder is full. Careful investigations may discover a plaque of multiple sclerosis or a disk lesion involving the spinal cord, but these are not always to be found, and the term *'detrusor instability'* is applied when no cause can be found.

If one can find the cause for an over-active spinal reflex treatment can be straightforward — e.g. the removal of a protruding intervertebral disc or tumour, but when, as is so often the case, no cause can be found, then

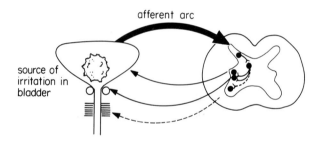

Fig. 13.4 Incontinence may be caused by irritation in the bladder from a stone or infection.

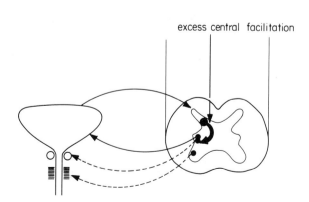

Fig. 13.5 Incontinence arising from excessive facilitation from higher centres.

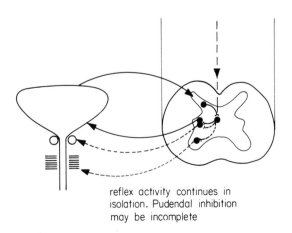

Fig. 13.6 Incontinence caused by absence of central inhibition due to disease in the spinal cord.

treatment is very unsatisfactory. Long-acting local anaesthetic or dilute phenol may be injected into the trigone at cystoscopy in the hope of blocking the afferent limb of the reflex arc; the nerves may be divided with a diathermy electrode introduced through the cystoscope — *bladder transection* — but the relief is seldom maintained.

An alternative technique is to add on to the bladder a generous patch of small bowel (Fig. 13.7) so that when the detrusor contracts, the pressure inside the bladder never rises so high that urine escapes (see p. 123). An alternative which is particularly useful when the bladder is very small is to enlarge it by means of the caecum — caecocystoplasty (see p. 153).

If the spinal cord is cut across above the level of the S2 and S3 segments by a bullet or a fracture of the cervical spine, the spinal centre is isolated from higher inhibition or facilitation, but its reflexes continue. In theory the bladder ought to empty out completely when it is full. In practice it does not do this because the spinal centre needs its higher connections for a fully coordinated reflex relaxation of the sphincter. No matter how forcefully the detrusor contracts, no matter how it hypertrophies, the failure of the sphincter to relax prevents complete emptying so that the bladder retains residual urine under high pressure which sooner or later becomes infected and leads to reflux and renal damage.

In incomplete lesions in the cord, e.g. in multiple sclerosis, similar

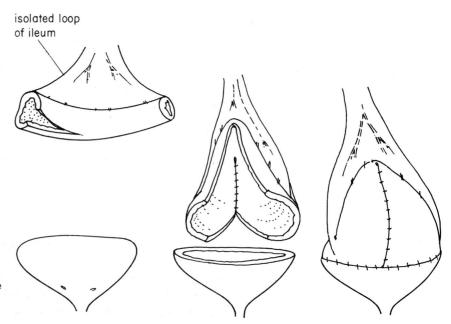

isolated loop
of ileum

Fig. 13.7 By adding on a patch formed from the small or large bowel the excess pressure inside the bladder is diminished.

disturbances of function are seen in different degrees of severity. Urodynamic tests again show a high pressure in the hypertrophied bladder, a low flow rate, and failure of the sphincter to relax.

Failure of the detrusor

The detrusor muscle may become paralysed either because the spinal centre is destroyed by a fracture at the level of T12 or L1, or because its connections with the bladder have been divided as a result of surgery in the pelvis, or because the nerve fibres have been stretched or have lost their insulating sheath as a result of diabetic neuropathy, a diagnosis which may need bladder evoked response studies (p. 130).

The result is that the bladder is converted into an inert bag which becomes larger and larger, without any increase in the pressure inside it. Eventually the huge flabby organ draws open the neck of the bladder and urine escapes — *overflow incontinence*. The danger is that the huge volume of urine sooner or later becomes infected.

Treatment of incontinence in the neuropathic bladder

The main danger is to the kidneys, when increased pressure inside the bladder is accompanied by urinary infection. For this reason, whether the neurological lesion results in an overactive or a paralysed detrusor, the aim of treatment is to ensure an empty low pressure bladder.

Intermittent self-catheterization

This is now the treatment of choice whenever it is practicable. If a patient passes a catheter on him or herself three or four times a day so emptying the bladder completely, urinary infection is negligible; if the patient does get an infection, the offending organism will usually be a harmless microbe to which he or she already has effective resistance.

If this is not practicable, a permanent indwelling catheter may be necessary.

Sphincterotomy

Some patients cannot manage to catheterize themselves, or when they can there is still a dangerously high pressure inside the bladder which threatens the kidneys. In men it is safer to keep the bladder empty at the expense of continence by cutting the internal and external sphincters with a diathermy knife introduced through a resectoscope — *sphincterotomy*

(Fig. 13.8). The male patient is then fitted with a *condom urinal* (Fig. 13.9) which fits the penis and collects urine into a bag worn on the leg. Condom urinals are always moist, and the skin tends to become irritated by the ammonia forming in the space between penis and condom. Buffered barrier creams help to reduce this soreness. These urinals tend

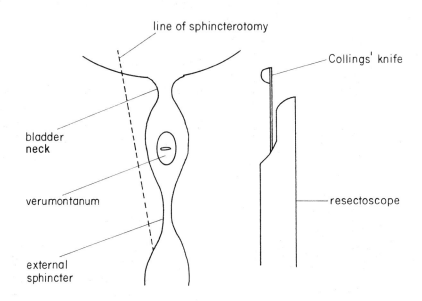

Fig. 13.8 Sphincterotomy: the internal and external sphincters are divided with a resectoscope knife.

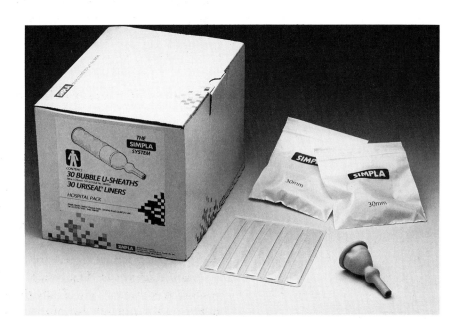

Fig. 13.9 A condom urinal.

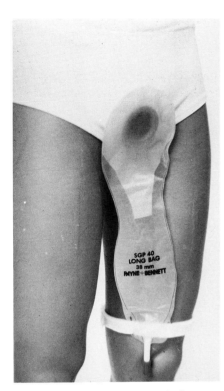

Fig. 13.10 A pubic pressure urinal.

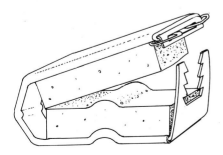

Fig. 13.11 The Cunningham clip.

to leak, especially at night. They must be changed daily after a wash or bath and careful drying. The manufacturer's instructions must be followed carefully if the patient is to obtain most benefit. It may be necessary to shave the part. Patients are tempted to put the retaining strap on too tightly with the result the foreskin may become oedematous and enlarged. Circumcision may make it possible to wear this kind of appliance.

Pubic pressure urinal

An alternative to the closely fitting condom urinal is the pubic pressure appliance (Fig. 13.10) where a loose cone that fits over the penis is held firmly against the symphysis pubis by tight underpants holding it over a ring on the base of the cone. The cone has a valve to stop urine leaking. Careful attention to fit, and washing and drying the area are essential.

Denervating the bladder

Unfortunately none of these incontinence appliances are suitable for women. If they can catheterize themselves, a persistently high pressure system may be converted into an atonic one by destroying the spinal nerve roots that convey impulses to and from the bladder. The S2 and S3 nerve roots may be cut at operation or injected with alcohol. Instead of being hypertrophied and overactive, the bladder is then converted into an inert bag, which the patient can keep empty by regular intermittent self-catheterization (see p. 188).

Mechanical devices for obtaining continence

DEVICES WORN EXTERNALLY

The most useful of all of these devices is the *Cunningham clip* (Fig. 13.11). It is placed across the penis in such a way that its sponge-rubber pads keep the urethra closed. The pressure needed to keep the urine from leaking out of the urethra is little less than that in its veins, so that there is always a risk of a pressure sore developing under the clip. Used carefully by intelligent men with normal penile sensation, it can be a most useful device; in others it can lead to disaster.

The *Edwards clip* (Fig. 13.12) has the same objective, to compress the urethra in women. It has all the drawbacks of the Cunningham clip, but again, if used carefully by informed women, can be helpful.

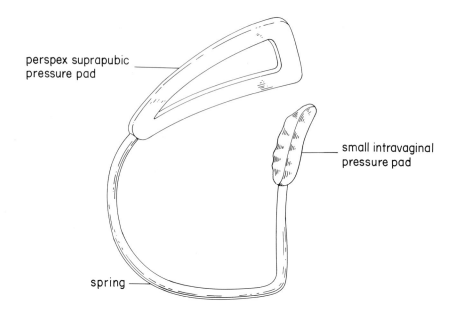

perspex suprapubic
pressure pad

small intravaginal
pressure pad

spring

Fig. 13.12 The Edwards clip.

DEVICES WORN INTERNALLY

Several of these have been introduced in recent years. The Scott inflatable device (Fig. 13.13) is a silicone rubber ballon shaped like a doughnut which is placed around the urethra which can be filled or emptied from a reservoir controlled by a tap placed in the scrotum (in men) or in the vulva (in women). When the patient wants to empty the bladder the balloon is deflated, and filled again when the bladder is empty. Practice is needed.

In *Kaufman's appliance* (Fig. 13.14) the ballon compresses the bulbar urethra all the time. The tension in the balloon must be just right, so that when the patient wants to void, he can strain just enough to overcome the extra resistance of the balloon.

These internal appliances are subject to the same inherent pitfalls as the external ones: the pressure needed to keep the urine in is very close to that in the urethral veins so pressure necrosis is very likely to occur. The implanted devices are wonders of modern plastics engineering, but they are also subject to mechanical failure, may need to be replaced and are exceedingly expensive. While they work, their happy owners are delighted, but they are apt to blame the surgeon when they fail.

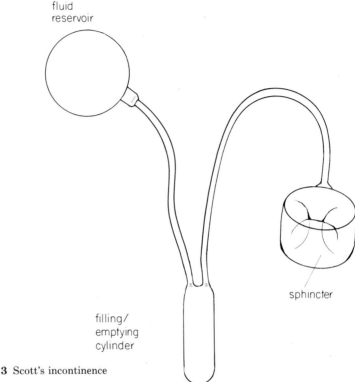

fluid
reservoir

filling/
emptying
cylinder

sphincter

Fig. 13.13 Scott's incontinence prosthesis.

Electrical stimulators

In some patients continence can be restored by faradic stimulation of the pelvic floor, either by externally applied electrodes — a method that is available in most departments of physiotherapy, or a small plug inserted into the anus or vagina and attached to a portable stimulator (Fig. 13.15). They have a very limited value except in some debilitated elderly patients who sometimes find that this stimulation helps to re-educate muscles which have become temporarily inactive.

NERVE ROOT STIMULATION

Recent developments have made it possible to implant tiny platinum electrodes housed in silicone directly onto the anterior roots of the S2 and S3 nerves. Stimulation of S2 empties the bladder and stimulation of S3 causes the sphincters to close off. The implants are controlled by a small radio transmitter carried by the patient. The early results are very promising.

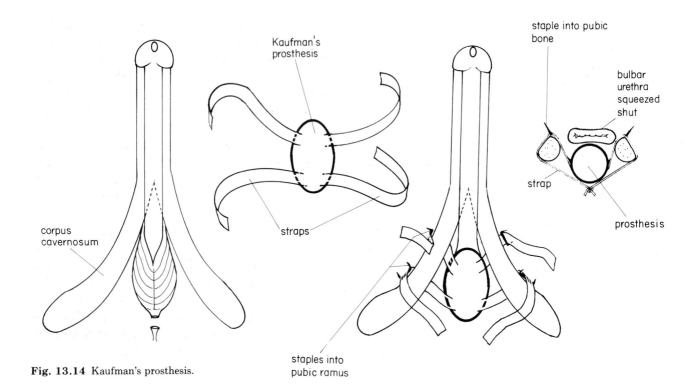

corpus
cavernosum

Kaufman's
prosthesis

straps

staple into pubic
bone

bulbar
urethra
squeezed
shut

strap

prosthesis

staples into
pubic ramus

Fig. 13.14 Kaufman's prosthesis.

Fig. 13.15 A vaginal stimulator.

Mechanical defects in the sphincter apparatus

Cut sphincters

The external sphincter apparatus may be accidentally cut during a prostatectomy. The diagnosis is sadly obvious when the urethra is examined endoscopically — there is a gap in what should be a complete ring of muscle (Fig. 13.16). A videocystogram may show that the patient is able to interrupt the flow of urine by contracting the voluntary striated muscles of his pelvic floor, but he cannot sustain this, since prolonged muscular contraction is a property of smooth rather than striated muscle.

The sphincter can also be injured in consequence of trauma, from a fractured pelvis, prolonged obstructed labour or surgical operations.

Displaced sphincters

Straining, coughing, laughing or lifting will raise the pressure inside the bladder, but normally two automatic safety mechanisms prevent urine from leaking.

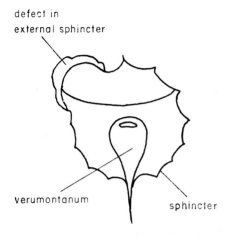

Fig. 13.16 An injured external sphincter seen through the resectoscope: a bite has been taken out of the ring of muscle at 10 o'clock.

1 There is a short length of urethra above the pelvic floor which is exposed to the intra-abdominal pressure: as it increases with a cough, so this short length of urethra is automatically squeezed by exactly the same amount (Fig. 13.17). In some women weakness in the pelvic floor allows the critical length of the urethra to prolapse down beyond the pelvic floor, where it is no longer automatically squeezed when intra-abdominal pressure is increased.

2 A reflex arc is called into play which increases the tone of the external sphincter whenever the intra-abdominal pressure is increased. Prolonged labour may damage the pudendal nerve through which this reflex is transmitted, a diagnosis that can only be made by studies of the bladder evoked response (p. 130)

As a result of either or both of these changes, women may leak urine each time they laugh, strain or cough. It is necessary to make sure that they are not suffering from an over-active detrusor whose contractions are being set off by increases in intra-abdominal pressure. This question is easily settled by a cystometrogram (see p. 126). If their detrusor is stable, and their stress incontinence solely due to mechanical displacement of the sphincter, then an operation to lift the bladder and urethra up into the abdomen will result in restoration of continence.

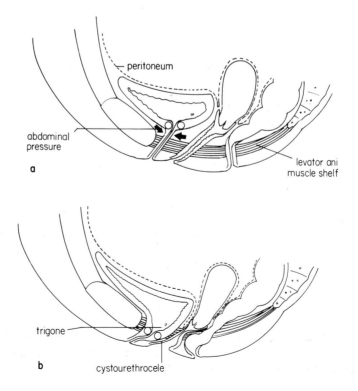

Fig. 13.17 The female perineal floor: (a) normal, and (b) in stress incontinence.

There are several ways of doing this:

1 *Anterior colporrhaphy.* Through a vaginal incision, the wall of the vagina is pleated under the urethra (Fig. 13.18).

2 *Stamey's suture.* The same end is achieved with a strong nylon suture passed down behind the symphysis and around the neck of the bladder — a safe operation particularly suited to elderly and debilitated women (Fig. 13.19).

3 *Marshall-Marchetti-Krantz operation.* Through an inconspicuous incision in the suprapubic crease the tissues either side of the urethra are sewn to the back of the symphysis pubis (Fig. 13.20).

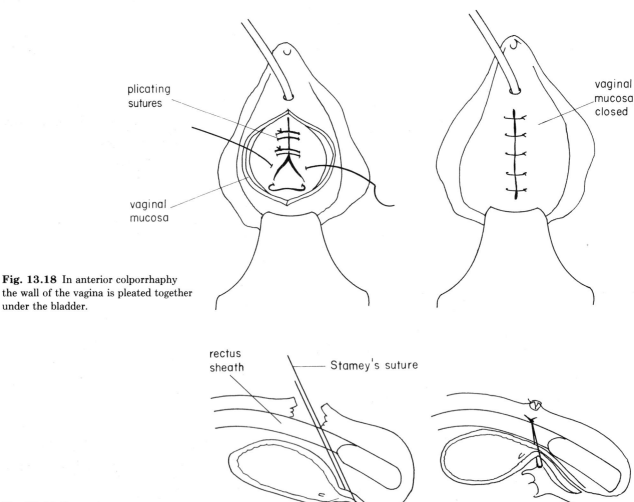

Fig. 13.18 In anterior colporrhaphy the wall of the vagina is pleated together under the bladder.

Fig. 13.19 Stamey's suture: a stout nylon suture is passed under the neck of the bladder to lift it up.

4 *Millin's sling.* Much the same result is achieved by passing a sling, made from rectus fascia or a synthetic material such as Marlex or nylon, under the urethra and bladder neck (Fig. 13.21).

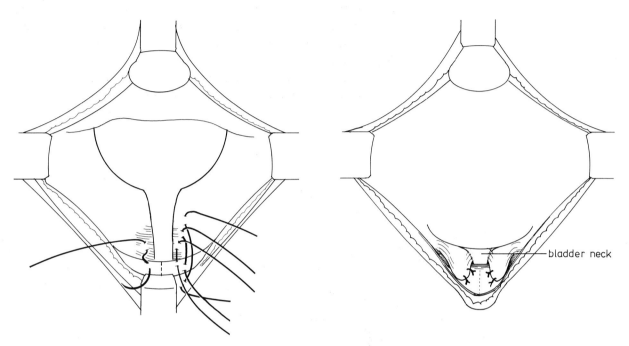

Fig. 13.20 Marshall–Marchetti–Krantz operation: through a retropubic incision the tissues either side of the urethra are sewn to the back of the symphysis pubis.

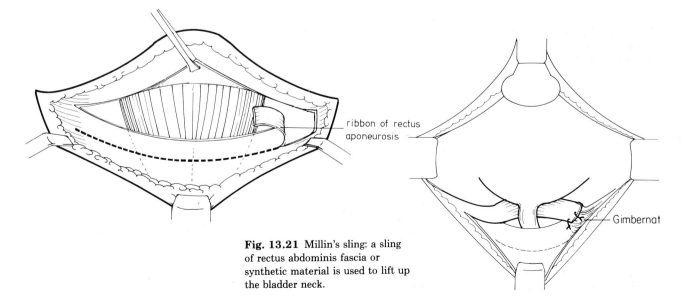

Fig. 13.21 Millin's sling: a sling of rectus abdominis fascia or synthetic material is used to lift up the bladder neck.

Preparation for operation

Except in the Stamey suture — which is a very minor procedure, the pre-operative preparation for the other operations includes a thorough pubic and perineal shave and evacuation of the bowel. If constipation leads to straining in the postoperative period the new supports of the urethra may give way.

Postoperative care

Many surgeons prefer the patient to rest in bed for several days. During this time leg exercises, supportive stockings and perhaps subcutaneous heparin may be given to prevent deep venous thrombosis, which is a common complication of these procedures.

A vaginal pack, if present, may be removed after 24 to 48 hours, and the catheter after about 10 days. Some surgeons prefer a suprapubic rather than a urethral catheter.

Before the catheter is removed the urine is cultured and any infection treated to avoid discomfort at a time when the patient needs to re-learn how to use her bladder. When the repair has been successful, the patient often has difficulty in voiding against the increased resistance at first, and it is quite usual to have to pass a catheter several times to make sure that the bladder is being emptied and to measure the volume of residual urine. Some surgeons prefer a suprapubic rather than a urethral catheter which can be clamped after 10 days and the result of the operation 'tried out' before the catheter is removed. If difficulty is experienced, it can easily be unclamped and reclamped later, so avoiding the repeated passing of a catheter. Occasionally it is necessary to teach a patient to catheterize herself for a week or two after she goes home (see p. 188).

Many of these patients will be mothers of young children, and some of the older women may live alone. It is a great temptation to pick up the toddler, carry the shopping, or get back to the housework. If the operation is to have a chance of success at least 6 weeks must go by before undue strain is placed on the scar that is to keep the repair permanently in position. It is important not only to make this clear to the patient, but also to see that adequate help is provided at home on discharge, or to ensure a period of convalescence away from the family.

Results

The result of all these repair operations for stress incontinence is about the same — about 80% do well, and 20% will fail. However a second attempt carries just as good a chance of succeeding, and so it is usual to start with the least invasive method.

Urinary diversion

It must be admitted that it is not always possible to achieve continence despite all these different techniques. For these patients the best that can be offered is a method of diversion of urine, whereby the urinary tract is artificially re-routed. The method that is offered must be adapted to the individual needs of the patient.

Ureterosigmoidostomy

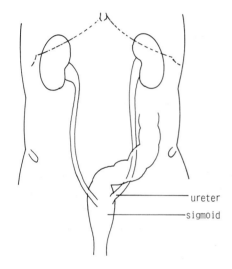

ureter
sigmoid

Fig. 13.22 Ureterosigmoidostomy.

Here the ureters are sewn into the sigmoid colon (Fig. 13.22). The urine collects in the rectosigmoid, and is passed like a fluid stool in the lavatory from time to time. When the patient has perfect control over the anal sphincters this can be acceptable, but one must first make sure of this by infusing 300 ml of saline into the rectum and getting the patient to walk about and cough. Few patients with a neuropathic bladder have adequate rectal control. There are also three long-term dangers of ureterosigmoid diversion.

1 *Infection* in the urine tracks up the ureters to the kidneys setting up intrarenal inflammation, scarring and often calculi.

2 *Reabsorption* of urine from the lumen of the colon is like giving the patient a continual dose of urine into his veins; the urea stimulates the tubules to force a diuresis. After a time the tubules become exhausted and unable to get rid of surplus acid and chloride resulting in uraemia and *hyperchloraemic acidosis*, for which sodium bicarbonate is given orally.

3 After a long time — 10 to 20 years — there is a risk of *cancer* in the sigmoid at the site of the implantation of the ureters, so all these patients must undergo regular colonoscopy.

The ileal conduit

This is the standard method of diversion after removal of the bladder for cancer (see p. 171). Its advantage is that urine does not linger in the lumen of the bowel and so hyperchloraemic acidosis is almost unknown. Although infection may occur, it is less serious because the pressure in the ileal conduit is low and damage to the kidneys and stone formation is less common. Nevertheless the patient pays a price for these advantages — the *adhesive urostomy appliance*.

No appliance will suit all patients all of the time. There are many alternatives and the patient must have the opportunity to handle and discuss the types available (see p. 173). Siting the stoma is no less important for a patient with incontinence than for one who has undergone total cystectomy for cancer, and those who are confined to a wheel chair have special difficulties. It is vital to ensure free drainage of urine in all positions as well as a system the patient is able to manage successfully. A piece of extra tubing attached to the outflow tap on certain appliances can, for instance, enable direct emptying into a lavatory pan.

Having chosen the optimum position, mark it clearly on the skin with indelible ink and send the chosen appliance to the operating theatre with the patient.

Psychological preparation

This is often more complex in younger men and women than in those undergoing cystectomy for cancer (see p. 171). Some find the idea of a *stoma* so revolting that they become profoundly depressed and anxious when faced with the idea of urinary diversion. Others are relieved after years of battling with an indwelling catheter. For everyone it is a change in the way they see themselves. Fortunately there are plenty who have successfully gone through the ordeal, many of whom are only too willing to give up a little of their time to explain how easy and convenient the arrangement can be. A few minutes of conversation with such a successful patient can give immense comfort and support to the frightened one facing an uncertain future.

Provided there is no other contraindication, there is no reason why *pregnancy*, with normal delivery or caesarian section should not be possible after urinary diversion, and there is no reason why it should give rise to *impotence* in men.

Diversion by an ileal conduit does not involve the removal of the bladder, and is less traumatic than diversion after cystectomy, but the patients are likely to be very dependent. Bowel preparation is more difficult as most patients with a neuropathic bladder also have a *neuropathic bowel* which makes them not only constipated but also to have little or no control. Diarrhoea before and after the operation may result in more time spent in bed with an increased risk of skin breakdown, chest infection and thrombosis, as well as mental stress.

Particularly when there has been long-term catheterization the *redundant bladder* left behind may fill with pus and produce an unpleasant discharge. Bladder washouts with chlorhexidine or normal saline may keep it under control but when the infection persists it may be necessary to cut the sphincters with a resectoscope (sphincterotomy), or make a small fistula between bladder and vagina to keep the bladder empty — a small operation but one that needs an anaesthetic.

Revision of the stoma

The stoma will be made to project just proud of the skin, so that it fits the opening of the appliance. As time goes by the bowel may elongate and the stoma protrude like a sausage into the lumen of the bag, where it may chafe and bleed. Occasionally when a patient puts on weight the stoma sinks in, making it difficult to fit an appliance. In either event the stoma may have to be revised, but this is seldom difficult.

Continent diversions

All of these are rather new and relatively untried. Any patient undergoing one of the newer continent diversions must understand its potential difficulties and complications and be prepared to undergo major surgery and still have some sort of appliance to manage.

The isolated rectosigmoid bladder

The ureters may be put into the sigmoid and the sigmoid cut across to make a urinary reservoir free of faecal contamination. The faeces are brought out through a colostomy (Fig. 13.23). It cannot be used after radiotherapy for cancer of the bladder because radiotherapy will have diminished the blood supply of the bowel, and it is no good for a patient who has imperfect control of a fluid stool — so that most patients with neuropathic bladders are excluded.

Continent intestinal pouches

Small or large bowel may be fashioned into a pouch capable of retaining a reasonable volume of urine. By forming a system of artificial valves, the urinary stoma is made so as not to leak, and the patient carries out intermittent catheterization through an inconspicuous hole — Kock's pouch (Fig. 13.24).

A similar type of pouch can be joined on to the urethra (Fig. 13.25) and if the urethral sphincter is not competent, an artificial inflatable sphincter may be placed around it.

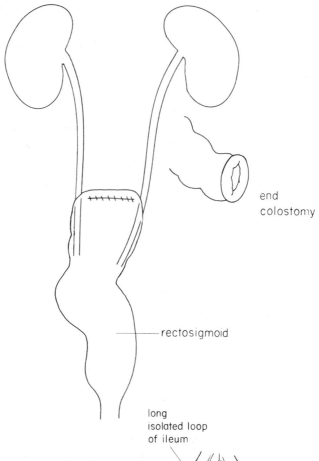

Fig. 13.23 The isolated rectosigmoid bladder: the ureters are put into the rectosigmoid so that continence is maintained by the anal sphincter. The faeces are diverted by an end colostomy.

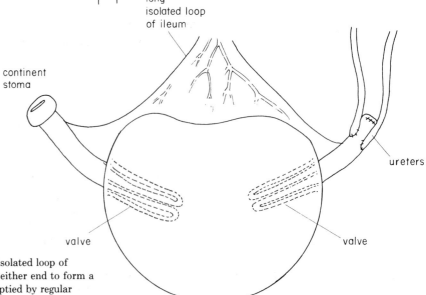

Fig. 13.24 Kock's continent pouch: a long isolated loop of ileum is made into a pouch, and invaginated either end to form a non-return valve. The continent pouch is emptied by regular self-catheterization.

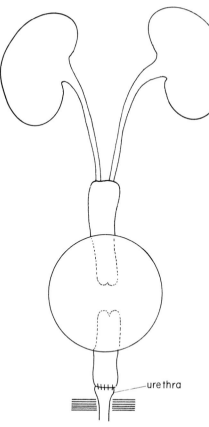

Fig. 13.25 A Kock's type of pouch may be anastomosed to the urethra.

Suprapubic cystostomy

This must be the oldest of all diversions, a tube in the bladder is used to collect urine (Fig. 13.26). The operation is very simple, but the same rules apply to a suprapubic cystostomy as to an ileal conduit — the tube must be placed where the patient can reach it and where scars and creases will not get in the way.

Today silicone rubber catheters are used which are non-irritant and the collecting bags are suspended from a waist belt which are more comfortable than bags attached to the leg. For permanent use there are certain disadvantages: the tip of the catheter may irritate the trigone and give pain in the tip of the penis which may set off reflex contractions of the detrusor. The catheters always get infected, and the bladders must be washed out regularly or stones will form.

After a time the Foley catheter can be exchanged for the simpler and smaller Malecot type of catheter (Fig. 13.27). This form of urinary diversion still has a place, albeit a limited one, in modern urology, and may be preferred by the sexually active man to a urethral catheter.

Vesicostomy

To avoid the discomfort and the risk of infection of a permanent suprapubic cystostomy, a tube may be made from the bladder to the surface in such a way that a catheter can be introduced, but urine does not leak out. The patient must pass a catheter at intervals. The opening of the tube may be placed near the base of the penis or the vulva so that the external opening can be quite inconspicuous (Fig. 13.28).

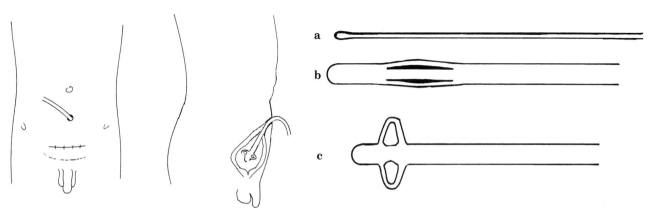

Fig. 13.26 Permanent suprapubic cystostomy.

Fig. 13.27 Malecot catheter used for permanent suprapubic drainage. (a) Introducer; (b) catheter stretched on introducer; (c) self-retaining 'wings' open.

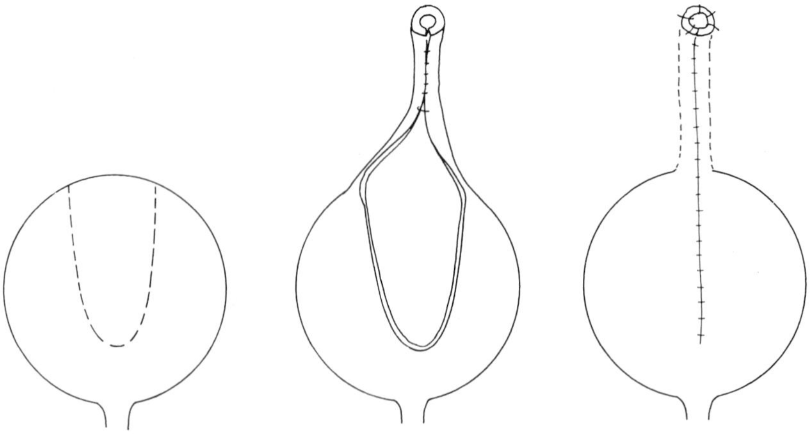

Fig. 13.28 Vesicostomy: a tube is made from the wall of the bladder and brought out on the skin where it can easily be catheterized.

Ureterostomy

The ureters may be brought to the skin and anastomosed in such a way that stenosis is avoided. Alternatively small tubes may be left indwelling and connected to a collecting bag (Fig. 13.29).

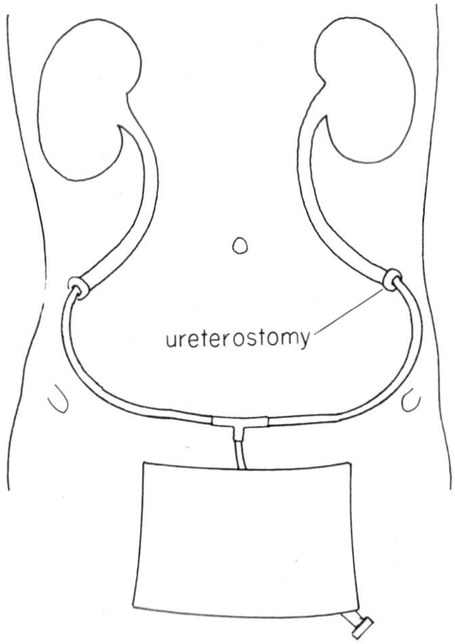

Caecocystoplasty

Not strictly a method of urinary diversion, nevertheless this is an operation with many features common to other techniques designed to form intestinal reservoirs. It is mainly used to enlarge the bladder when it has become shrunken as a result of the scarring that follows treatment of tuberculosis (see p. 52) and in bladders that are so severely inflamed and painful that they cannot retain more than a tiny quantity of urine — a condition seen in certain forms of chronic cystitis including Hunner's ulcer or interstitial cystitis (see p. 165). The principle of the operation is quite simple — a segment of ileum and caecum is isolated from the bowel on its own mesentery (Fig. 13.30). The ileum is anastomosed to the ascending colon to restore continuity, and then the caecum is turned upside down and sewn on to the bladder (Fig. 13.31).

Particular pre- and postoperative care

Before operation it is necessary to explain the need for careful and effective bowel clearance. The continuity of the bowel will be restored and patients are unlikely to notice any disturbance of function after recovering from the operation. (Since the appendix will also be removed, they are spared the future risk of appendicitis.)

Different surgeons prefer different methods of bowel preparation, but

Fig. 13.29 When the ureters are of normal calibre, small tubes may be left indwelling and joined by a T-connection to a bag suspended from the waist.

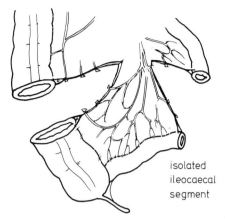

Fig. 13.30 Caecocystoplasty: a length of terminal ileum, caecum and ascending colon is isolated on its own mesentery.

in general bowel preparation will include aperients, enemata, washouts and possibly antibiotics to sterilize the colon. A fluid diet is usual for 2 to 3 days. During this period of preparation the diarrhoea adds to the patient's discomfort. He or she must also be prepared for several days of intravenous therapy and nasogastric aspiration during the period of paralytic ileus. There will also be drains at the site of the bowel and bladder anastomoses; the quantity and type of drainage can be measured and assessed if tube drains are used, connected to drainage bags. The drains are shortened after 5 or 6 days, and removed when drainage is minimal. The bowel should not be allowed to become overdistended, a flatus tube should be passed when necessary.

After the operation there will be suprapubic and urethral catheters in the newly constructed bladder to keep it empty while healing takes place. The lining of the caecum continues to secrete mucus, so these catheters must be large ones if they are not to become blocked.

Gently milking the catheters when mucus appears helps to keep them patent. If there is an excess of mucus 1.4% sodium bicarbonate solution may be run in through the suprapubic catheter and out through the urethral one, never using any force. A high fluid intake, at first intravenous, and later by mouth, helps to wash away this mucus in the flow of urine.

The appearance of mucus in the urine is unpleasant, and some people find it worrying; assure them that it is normal. Patients take a little while to get used to a strange sensation when emptying the bladder and at first it is helpful to void at regular intervals rather than wait for the desire to pass urine. Control of urination is usually good during the daytime but at

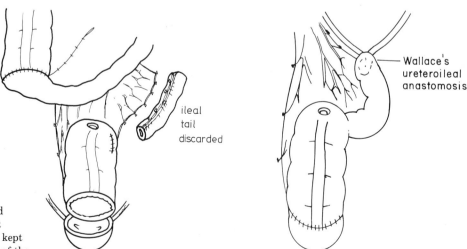

Fig. 13.31 The caecum is inverted and anastomosed to the opened-out bladder: the terminal ileum may be kept or removed, according to the needs of the individual patient.

night the new bladder, which is now made almost entirely out of caecum, may empty of its own accord. This bedwetting will cause distress in the first few weeks after operation if patients have not been warned to expect it, and supplied with appropriate incontinence pads. You can reassure them that this unpleasant complication will soon cease.

They also need to be warned that because their new bladder is made of large intestine it will contract if stimulated with the kind of purgatives that act upon the large bowel — e.g. senna and cascara so that if in the future they suffer from constipation they should seek relief in bran and bulk laxatives.

Further reading

Ashken, M. H., Abrams, P. H. & Lawrence, W. T. (1984) Stamey endoscopic bladder neck suspension for stress incontinence. *British Journal of Urology*, **56**, 629–634.

Blackford, H. N., Murray, K., Stephenson, T. P. & Mundy, A. R. (1984) Results of transvesical infiltration of the pelvic plexuses with phenol in 116 patients. *British Journal of Urology*, **56**, 647–649.

Blandy, J. P. (1986) *Operative Urology*, 2nd edn. Blackwell Scientific Publications, Oxford.

Brocklehurst, J. C. (ed.) (1984) *Medicine in Old Age: Urology in the Elderly.* Churchill Livingstone, Edinburgh.

Duckett, J. W. & Caldamone, A. A. (1985) Congenital disorders of the bladder. In *Textbook of Genito-Urinary Surgery*, vol. 1, eds Whitfield, H. N. & Hendry, W. F., pp. 178–202. Churchill Livingstone, Edinburgh.

Ewing, R., Choa, B. & Shuttleworth, K. E. D. (1983) Pelvic evoked responses. *British Journal of Urology*, **55**, 639–641.

Feneley, R. C. L. & Blannin, J. P. (1984) *Incontinence.* Patient Handbook No. 18. Churchill Livingstone, Edinburgh.

Griffiths, D. J. (1980) *Urodynamics.* Medical Physics Handbooks No. 4. Adam Hilger, Bristol.

McGuire, E. J., Lytton, B., Pepe, V., & Kohorn, E. I. (1976) Stress urinary incontinence. *Obstetrics and Gynecology*, **47**, 255–264.

Mandelstam, D. (Ed.) (1980) *Incontinence and its Management.* Croom Helm, London.

Mandelstam, D. (1984) Incontinence — re-education of the pelvic floor. *Nursing, 2nd Series*, **29**, 867–868.

Shepherd, A. M., Blannin, J. P. & Feneley, R. C. L. (1982) Changing attitudes in the management of urinary incontinence — the need for specialist nursing. *British Medical Journal*, **284**, 645–646.

Stephenson, T. P. & Mundy, A. R. (1985) Treatment of the neuropathic bladder by enterocystoplasty and selective sphincterotomy or sphincter ablation and replacement. *British Journal of Urology*, **57**, 27–31

Swash, M. (1985) New concepts in incontinence. *British Medical Journal*, **290**, 4–5.

Tiptaft, R. C., Woodhouse, C. R. J. & Badenoch, D. F. (1984) Mazindol for nocturnal enuresis. *British Journal of Urology*, **56**, 641–643.

Turner-Warwick, R. T. & Whiteside, C. G. (1979) Clinical urodynamics. *Urological Clinics of North America*, **6**, 1–304.

White, H. M. (1984) Aids to continence — simple and sophisticated. *Nursing 2nd Series*, **29**, 855–858.

Whitaker, R. H. (1985) Artificial urinary sphincters. *British Medical Journal*, **290**, 1927–1928.

14 *The bladder — benign conditions*

Congenital anomalies of the bladder

Exstrophy

Babies may be born with a defect in the lower part of the abdominal wall which is due to the development of an abnormally large cloacal membrane in the fetus, which, when it dissolves, leaves a triangular gap in which the raw bladder is exposed (Fig. 14.1) — *exstrophy.*

These babies should be referred at once to a specialist paediatric urological centre where early repair may result in almost normal function,

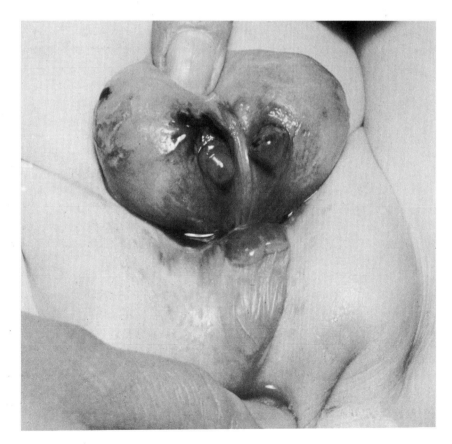

Fig. 14.1 Exstrophy.

although it may take several operations to achieve continence. Whenever possible parents should be encouraged to share in caring. Secure dressings, restraints and things to occupy the child are important while healing is taking place.

Epispadias

This is a lesser version of this condition in which the urethra opens out on the top of a short stumpy penis (Fig. 14.2). To get a good result from surgical repair is very difficult. As with exstrophy these babies should be referred to centres where the surgeons see enough cases to allow them to develop a standard and successful technique. The sooner they are referred the better the result.

Trauma to the bladder

Closed injuries usually occur in patients with a distended bladder who suffer an abdominal injury — classically the drunk who gets run over (Fig. 14.3). The distended bladder may burst into or outside of the peritoneal cavity — intra- or extraperitoneal rupture. Observation and treatment for other multiple injuries is generally required.

Intraperitoneal rupture

It is easy to miss this injury because at first the urine is not very irritating to the peritoneum. All suspect patients must be admitted for observation,

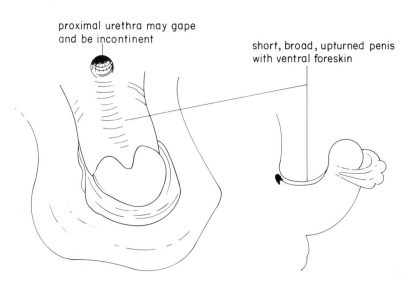

proximal urethra may gape and be incontinent

short, broad, upturned penis with ventral foreskin

Fig. 14.2 Epispadias: the typical deformity.

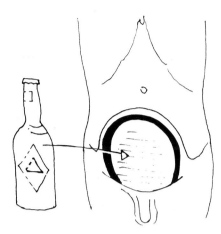

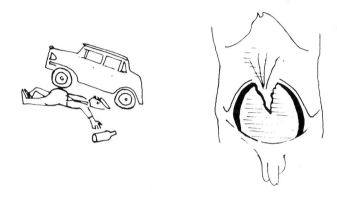

Fig. 14.3 Closed injury of the bladder is usually seen in a drunk who has a full bladder at the time of injury.

their abdominal girth is measured and regular attempts are made to hear bowel sounds. A cystogram will confirm the leakage. When the leak is small it can be managed by an indwelling catheter. Only in rare and neglected cases is laparotomy needed to evacuate a large accumulation of stale or infected urine from the peritoneal cavity and close the laceration in the bladder.

Extraperitoneal rupture

Extraperitoneal rupture of the bladder may complicate fracture of the pelvis. It is usually managed by simple suprapubic drainage in the acute stage of the injury.

Penetrating injuries

Penetrating injuries of the bladder are found at laparotomy for penetrating abdominal knife or bullet injuries. The bladder heals very well if it is simply sewn up and drained with an indwelling catheter for 7 to 10 days.

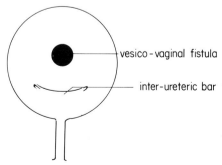

Iatrogenic injury of the bladder

The bladder may be injured in operations to remove the rectum or uterus. At hysterectomy if the cervix of the uterus is firmly attached to the bladder a hole is easily made just above the trigone — *vesicovaginal fistula* (Fig. 14.4). It is usually the patient who first notices that fluid is running away from her vagina 5 to 10 days after hysterectomy. Nowadays, after confirming that the fluid is indeed urine (by measuring its creatinine) the fistula is closed without delay.

Fig. 14.4 Post-hysterectomy vesicovaginal fistula as it appears at cystoscopy.

Closure of vesicovaginal fistula

Under general anaesthesia cystoscopy is performed to show the hole between the bladder and the vagina. At the same time ureterograms are performed on either side to make sure that neither ureter has been injured as well.

Small vesicovaginal fistulae are easily closed from the vaginal approach: a small Foley catheter is put in the hole, the balloon blown up and the fistula drawn down so that it can be easily seen, excised and closed off (Fig. 14.5). Unfortunately most fistulae are large and placed too high up to allow a vaginal approach.

Through the abdominal incision originally used for the hysterectomy, the bladder is divided down to the fistula (Fig. 14.6) and dissected off the vagina. After closing the hole in the vagina it is covered with omentum (Fig. 14.7) and then the bladder is closed. Temporary splints may be left in the ureters and a catheter is left in the bladder.

The nursing care is the same as after repair of an injured ureter (see p. 112)

Postpartum vesicovaginal fistula

This is an entirely different condition which is today only seen in countries lacking obstetric services. It is caused by obstructed labour that is so prolonged that ischaemic necrosis develops to involve the neck of the bladder and the urethra in a gigantic pressure sore (Fig. 14.8). The mother

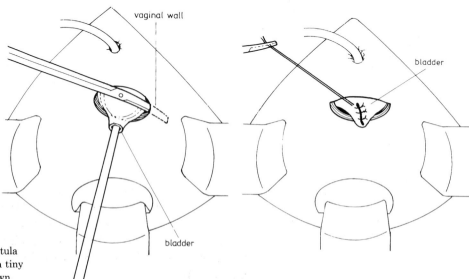

vaginal wall

bladder

bladder

Fig. 14.5 A small vesicovaginal fistula may be closed through the vagina; a tiny Foley catheter brings the fistula down.

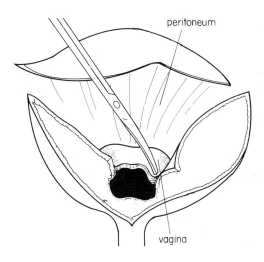

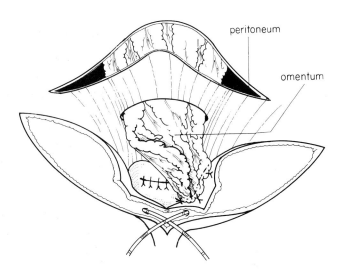

Fig. 14.6 Operation for a large postoperative vesicovaginal fistula: the bladder is bisected down to the fistula and separated from the wall of the vagina.

Fig. 14.7 After closing the hole in the vagina it is covered with a plug of omentum.

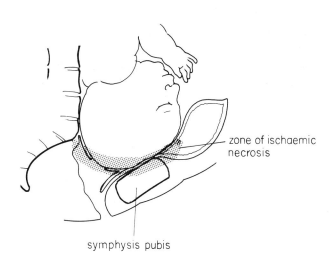

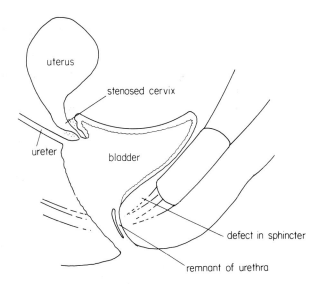

Fig. 14.8 Vesicovaginal fistula after prolonged neglected labour: (a) pressure of the fetal head against the pubis leads to ischaemic necrosis of the floor of the bladder, and (b) when the dead tissue finally separates there is a large defect.

is fortunate to survive with her life, the baby always dies. It takes months before the dead tissue has separated and the secondary infection has come under control. Repairing these fistulae is exceedingly difficult for in addition to closing the defect in the bladder it is necessary to try to reconstruct its sphincter. One method makes use of a graft of the gracilis muscle (Fig. 14.9).

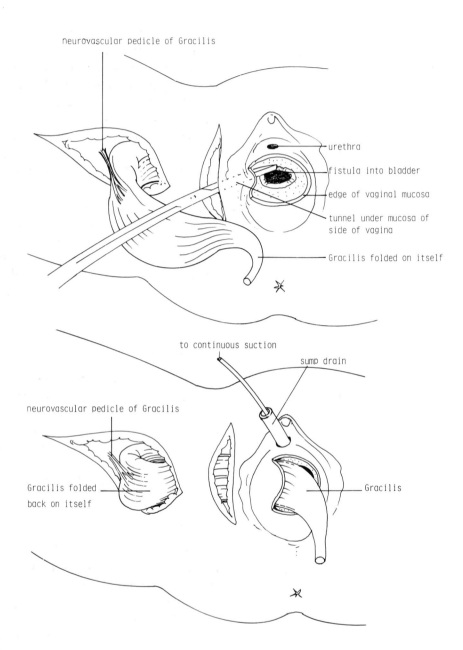

neurovascular pedicle of Gracilis

urethra

fistula into bladder

edge of vaginal mucosa

tunnel under mucosa of side of vagina

Gracilis folded on itself

to continuous suction

sump drain

neurovascular pedicle of Gracilis

Gracilis folded back on itself

Gracilis

Fig. 14.9 Repair of a large vesicovaginal fistula using the gracilis muscle.

Inflammation of the bladder

Acute cystitis

Acute cystitis is very common in women about 70% of whom will experience one or more attacks sooner or later. Bacteria enter the bladder along the urethra and multiply in the urine. At first only the lining urothelium of the urethra and bladder is inflamed, later on the inflammation may extend more deeply into the wall of the bladder.

The organisms responsible for acute cystitis are generally those which normally inhabit the intestine, e.g. *Escherischia coli, Klebsiella, Proteus mirabilis* and *Streptococcus faecalis.* In patients who have been given antibiotics, and especially those who have been in hospital for any time, the normal bowel flora is contaminated with resistant strains of organisms especially *Pseudomonas pyocyanea* and *Acinetobacter.*

The symptoms of cystitis begin with irritation in the urethra, but soon the patient has a strong desire to pass urine every few minutes; only small amounts of urine are passed with stinging pain and perhaps a little blood. The pain may be felt in the suprapubic region and in the perineum.

The inflammation may spread up to the ureters and kidneys causing pain in the iliac fossae and loins, and if it involves the renal parenchyma the bacteria may get into the bloodstream and give rise to fever, rigors and septicaemia (see p. 48).

Investigations

In women cystitis is so common and usually so harmless, that extensive investigations in a single attack are seldom justified. In males, on the contrary, cystitis may signify some serious underlying abnormality in the urinary system — e.g. residual urine or a stone. In either sex repeated episodes of cystitis call for an IVU to exclude such abnormalities and if there has been haematuria, then cystoscopy is always performed, once the infection is under control, to rule out cancer of the bladder.

Treatment

Ideally, one should culture the urine so that the antibiotic can be prescribed according to the sensitivity of the organism, but in practice, since this may delay treatment the antimicrobial that is most likely to be appropriate is usually given, changing it later if necessary when the bacteriological sensitivities have been reported on.

More important than the treatment of these infections is their prevention. The bladder is like a dustbin. To keep it clean it must be emptied out frequently. A patient who is prone to repeated episodes of urinary infection must train herself to pass urine at least every 2 hours and keep the system well washed out by getting into the habit of drinking a glass (250 ml) of fluid no less often. By these means the bacteria never get enough time to breed in the bladder and most attacks can be prevented.

However, when resistance is low, e.g. after influenza, the occasional relapse will still occur and the patient will need antibiotics. The patient is provided with a reserve supply of a safe antibiotic such as trimethoprim, nalidixic acid, nitrofurantoin or a sulphonamide and advised to start taking them at the first inkling that another infection has started: 24 to 48 hours is long enough in most cases.

During the attack of cystitis passing urine can be exceedingly painful and this discomfort can be lessened by making the urine alkaline with oral sodium bicarbonate or citrate, but this of course does not kill the bacteria.

Chronic cystitis

Most patients have repeated attacks of acute cystitis rather than a deep seated chronic infection of the wall of the bladder, but this does occur especially in elderly women. A cystoscopy will usually show that the wall of the bladder is studded with collections of lymphocytes under the urothelium which signify a long history of repeated infections. Patients with such an established infection need very prolonged courses of antibiotics before they get better. The causative organism is usually an ordinary *E. coli* but two other more serious types of chronic infection must be noted: *tuberculosis* and *schistosomiasis.*

Tuberculosis

Tuberculosis is always suspected when the urine contains pus but no obvious bacteria *sterile pyuria.* Cystoscopy may reveal oedema, ulcers or the typically deformed ureteric orifice, and biopsy may provide the diagnosis. It is always secondary to tuberculosis in the kidney (see p. 52). When it heals the bladder may contract so much that it may have to be enlarged by the operation of caecocystoplasty (see p. 153).

Schistosomiasis

This is one of the most important and most common of all the diseases of the modern world, affecting millions of people in Egypt, Iraq, Africa, the West Indies and Brazil. It is caused by a little flatworm — *Schistosoma* (Fig. 14.10) which lives inside human veins, attached to the lining of the vein by a sucker. The male fluke enfolds the female in a long slit down the front of his body (Greek, *schisto* = split, *soma* = body). The worms were first discovered by Theodor Bilharz, a German pathologist, when working in Cairo — hence the disease is often called *bilharziasis.*

A favourite place for these worms to take up residence is in the veins just under the lining of the bladder. As the mother fluke lays her eggs (Fig. 14.11) they bore through the lining of the bladder and float off in the urine. When the patient passes water into a slow-moving stream or irrigating canal the eggs hatch out and tiny hairy creatures — *miracidia* — emerge and swim about until they find a nearby unsuspecting snail into which they penetrate, grow and divide to form a cystic structure from which finally emerge the next generation of tiny flukes — the *cercariae*. These leave the snail and swim about waiting for the next human being to put a toe into the water.

It only takes 10 seconds of contact with water infested with cercariae for a patient to be infected by them: they pass through the skin into the lymphatics, giving rise to a local rash — 'swimmers itch'. From the lymphatics they reach the bloodstream, causing a fever as they are carried all round the body, until they find a partner, marry and settle down in a convenient vein. The pairs of *Schistosoma* flukes find the most desirable residences in the veins of the pelvic organs, especially the bladder and rectosigmoid and it is here that the infestation is most profuse and does most damage.

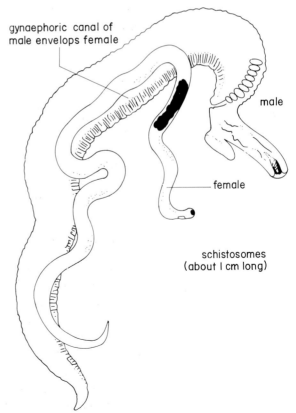

Fig. 14.10 A pair of *Schistosoma* flatworms: each about 0.5 cm long.

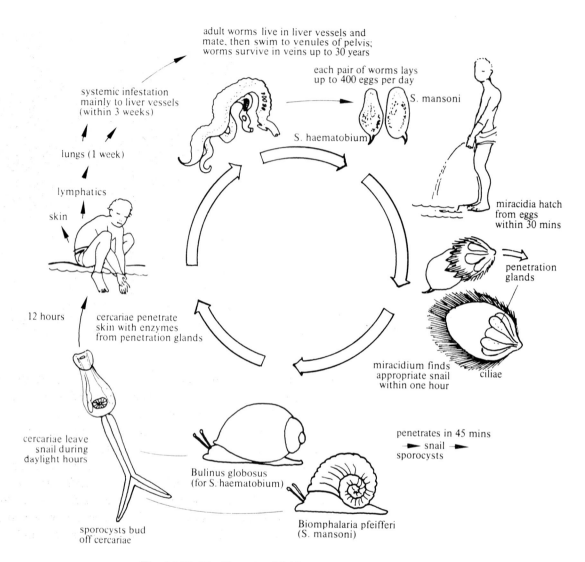

adult worms live in liver vessels and mate, then swim to venules of pelvis; worms survive in veins up to 30 years

each pair of worms lays up to 400 eggs per day

S. mansoni

S. haematobium

systemic infestation mainly to liver vessels (within 3 weeks)

lungs (1 week)

lymphatics

skin

miracidia hatch from eggs within 30 mins

penetration glands

12 hours

cercariae penetrate skin with enzymes from penetration glands

miracidium finds appropriate snail within one hour

ciliae

penetrates in 45 mins
snail sporocysts

cercariae leave snail during daylight hours

Bulinus globosus (for S. haematobium)

Biomphalaria pfeifferi (S. mansoni)

sporocysts bud off cercariae

Fig. 14.11 The life-cycle of *Schistosoma*.

As the eggs work their way through the wall of the bladder they give rise to haematuria. Cystoscopy shows the characteristic shiny eggs under the urothelium, looking like grains of sand: later on they cause ulceration and polypi and in the end the patient develops cancer (see p. 167).

So many eggs are present in the wall of the bladder in some of these patients that their calcified shadows can outline the bladder in the X-ray as if traced with chalk (Fig. 14.12).

Schistosomiasis can only be prevented by the most basic of public health measures, keeping sewage out of the drinking water. But in parts of

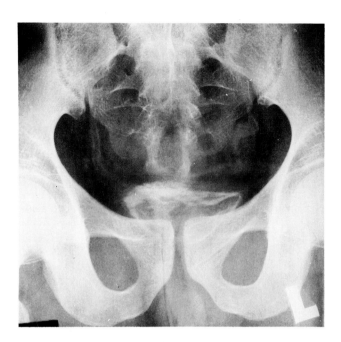

Fig. 14.12 Calcification in the wall of the bladder caused by the reaction around innumerable dead schistosoma eggs.

the world where schistosomiasis is most common, this is often very difficult. One might think that to keep urine and faeces out of the drinking water supply would need only the elementary latrines — holes in the ground, but this is not so simple in areas where the water table is within inches of the surface as it is in much of the Nile delta.

The least relevant treatment is to attack the living worms in the patient by giving drugs. Niridazole and metrifonate given together in a single dose or in short courses may be very effective, but for the peasant who is obliged to return to the fields to earn his living standing up to his knees in water teeming with cercariae such medication is futile.

Hunner's ulcer — interstitial cystitis

A curious chronic inflammatory change occurs in the wall of the bladder, usually in women, whose cause is unknown. The process extends right through the wall of the bladder. The patients have such severe frequency and such intense pain whenever the shrunken bladder is full that they can be socially crippled.

A biopsy confirms the diagnosis. Treatment is unsatisfactory: for a time there may be prolonged relief if the bladder is overdistended under general anaesthesia. Sometimes 50 ml of dimethylsulphoxide (DMSO) instilled into the bladder every few weeks will make life tolerable, even though it hurts for an hour or two. Eventually it may be necessary to re-move the bladder and replace it with caecum — *caecocystoplasty* (see p. 153).

Further reading

Blandy, J. P. (1989) *Lecture Notes on Urology*, 4th edn. Blackwell Scientific Publications, Oxford.

Blandy, J. P. (1986) *Operative Urology*, 2nd edn. Blackwell Scientific Publications, Oxford.

Duckett, J. W. & Caldamone, A. A. (1985) Congenital disorders of the bladder. In *Textbook of Genito-Urinary Surgery*, vol. 1, Eds Whitfield, H. N. & Hendry, W. F., pp. 178-202. Churchill Livingstone, Edinburgh.

Smith, D. R. (1984) Disorders of the bladder, prostate and seminal vesicles. In *General Urology*, ed. Smith, D. R., pp. 524-538. Lange, Los Altos, California.

15 *The bladder — cancer*

This is a very common disease all over the world. In Egypt and Africa it follows infestation with schistosomiasis, in Europe it is associated with industrial agents, particularly in the chemical and rubber industry, and above all *smoking* — which is one of the most important causes of bladder cancer today. This must be spelt out, especially to the younger patients, to help them kick the habit.

The first sign is usually painless haematuria. Any haematuria must always be investigated as early as possible by IVU and cystoscopy. The blood loss may be so severe and prolonged as to cause anaemia and require transfusion.

Pathology

Most bladder cancers arise from the normal lining of the bladder, the urothelium: but like any other specialized epithelium it can change in response to repeated irritation and come to resemble skin if repeatedly irritated by a stone or chronic infection such as schistosomiasis, and give rise to a *squamous cell carcinoma*. Metaplasia may also change the urothelium into something like that of the bowel which may give rise to an *adenocarcinoma*.

In the usual *urothelial carcinoma* the outlook for the patient depends on the grade of malignancy (G1, G2 and G3) and on how deeply the cancer has penetrated into the wall of the bladder — the *pathological stage* (Fig. 15.1).

Before the cancer eats into the muscle of the bladder (T1) the outlook is good. Once the muscle is invaded (T2, T3 and worse) the outlook is worse unless treatment is very energetic, because in the muscle there are many lymphatics and once into them the tumour cells may be spread widely.

The diagnosis and assessment of a bladder tumour is made by cystoscopy, biopsy and examination under anaesthesia which gives the grade and stage of the tumour. At this cystoscopy all tumours that are superficial, i.e. have not invaded the muscle are removed by transurethral resection.

Superficial cancers

Transurethral resection of a bladder tumour (TURBT)

The patient is prepared for general or spinal anaesthesia and the possible need for an indwelling catheter and bladder irrigation afterwards is explained.

Under general or spinal anaesthesia a *resectoscope* is passed into the bladder. Its semicircular diathermy loop cuts out long strips of tissue taking first the 'bush' of the cancer (Fig. 15.2) and then the 'stalk' (Fig. 15.3), the specimens being carefully labelled. The stalk will be examined to see whether muscle has been invaded, for if so, then the patient will need some additional treatment (Fig. 15.4).

If the resection has been extensive analgesia such as pethidine may be needed postoperatively, always bearing in mind the possibility of clot retention or extravasation of urine, and the need to make sure that the catheter is draining freely.

Before discharge, the patient must be warned that some bleeding is to be expected about 10 to 14 days after operation, due to the separation of the scab inside the bladder. Increasing their fluid intake is all that is usually necessary to wash the blood out and prevent it from clotting. This secondary haemorrhage is more likely to occur in the presence of infection so that mid-stream urine must be cultured, the result checked and appropriate antibiotics provided if necessary.

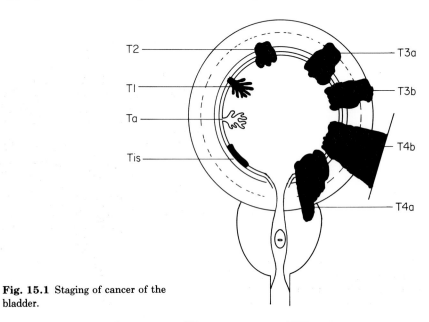

Fig. 15.1 Staging of cancer of the bladder.

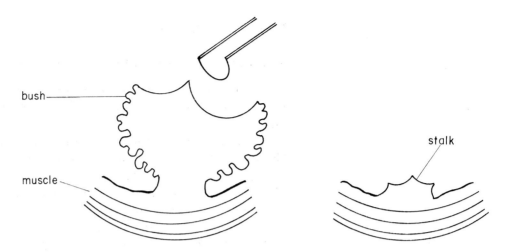

Fig. 15.2 Transurethral resection of a bladder tumour: first the 'bush' is removed.

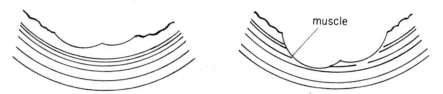

Fig. 15.3 The 'stalk' is removed separately to see if the tumour has invaded the muscle of the bladder wall.

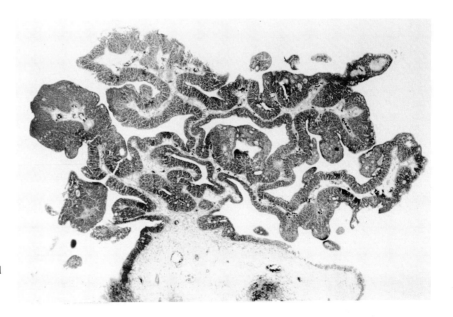

Fig. 15.4 Histological section through bladder tumour removed by transurethral resection showing muscle from which the stage is assessed.

Even when the tumours are superficial (T1) the patient is kept under regular cystoscopic review — at first every three months and the need for this must be explained to the patient. It sometimes helps them to think of them as little 'warts' which tend to come back again and again — easy to deal with when they form only a tiny recurrence, but if neglected and allowed to reach the stage where they are invasive, then they require much more extensive treatment.

Often the tumours are multiple or return in large numbers very quickly. One may slow them up by *intravesical chemotherapy* with various 'adjuvant agents' — Thiotepa, Epodyl, Adriamycin, Mitomycin, or BCG which are all successful for some tumours some of the time, but none of them work for all of them all of the time.

Intravesical chemotherapy

The technique of intravesical medication is simple but it needs care to achieve the maximum therapeutic effect, and strict precautions in the handling of these cytotoxic drugs must be observed.

The patient may have difficulty holding his urine, so that fluid intake should be reduced for 2 to 3 hours beforehand, and diuretics withheld. There may already be an indwelling catheter, otherwise a Jaques or Foley catheter is passed and the bladder emptied. The drug of choice in a volume of 30 to 50 ml is then injected gently and the catheter removed or clamped off, according to instructions. The drug should be kept in the bladder for at least 30 minutes and up to an hour if possible before being passed or drained out.

Side-effects

All of these drugs can have side-effects. With Thiotepa there is a risk that the drug may be absorbed and poison the bone marrow leading to a deficit in white cells — leukopaenia — and patients die from the effects of bacterial infection which they would normally have been able to resist. With Adriamycin and Epodyl, the lining of the bladder may be so irritated that the patient suffers pain and frequency from chemical cystitis. With Mitomycin, droplets spilt on the skin when the drug is injected into the bladder, may give rise to a severe skin hypersensitivity reaction. BCG may cause a form of tuberculosis that requires treatment with chemotherapy. The addition of these intravesical agents to regular cystoscopic control can allow the patient to keep his bladder for many years. Only when these treatments fail, need the bladder be removed by *total cystectomy.*

Invasive cancers — T2, T3, etc.

When the cancer is invading the muscle of the bladder (Fig. 15.5) there are today three choices of treatment: (1) immediate total cystectomy, (2) preoperative radiotherapy followed by planned cystectomy, and (3) radiotherapy alone, reserving 'salvage' cystectomy for those cases where radiotherapy has failed.

1 *Total cystectomy* may be performed without any preliminary radiotherapy. This has the advantage that the difficulty and danger of the operation is somewhat less, and it may be possible to provide a continent form of urinary diversion since the intestine has not been irradiated (see below).

2 By giving preoperative *radiotherapy* a few days or weeks before the cystectomy it is hoped that cancer cells just beyond the limit of surgical removal of the bladder may be killed. A lower dose of radiation is given than in the third option, so that the cystectomy is not made more hazardous and the option to offer a continent form of diversion is still available.

3 *Radiotherapy and salvage cystectomy.* In this system (which is used in our Hospital) a course of *radical radiotherapy* is given over a period of 6 weeks with a *linear accelerator* (Fig. 15.6).

This may cause temporary 'irradiation cystitis', i.e. frequency and discomfort and the haematuria may persist. The patient needs as much support as possible. With the necessity of having to travel for treatment, tiredness, lack of sleep, nausea, loss of appetite and diarrhoea, it is difficult not to be discouraged. It will help to explain that the symptoms

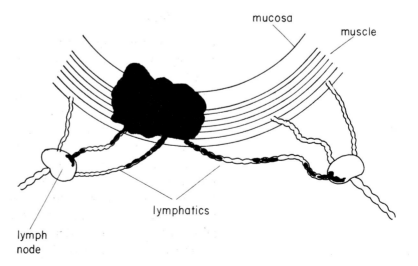

Fig. 15.5 Once the cancer invades the muscle of the bladder it can spread via lymphatics, and local treatment is no longer enough.

often get worse before they get better. Explanatory handouts to take home are invaluable, stressing the need to report problems so that symptomatic relief can be instituted quickly.

Over half the invasive bladder cancers will respond completely to radiation and the cancer will disappear completely within 3 to 6 months of the end of the course of treatment, and when it does respond like this there is an excellent chance of a permanent cure.

Unfortunately in the other half the tumour does not go away, or continues to grow and then the bladder has to be removed by the operation of *radical total cystectomy* provided the patient is well enough to undergo this operation. If complete removal is not possible it may still be a kindness to carry out a 'palliative' urinary diversion with an ileal loop, to relieve uncontrollable pain and frequency.

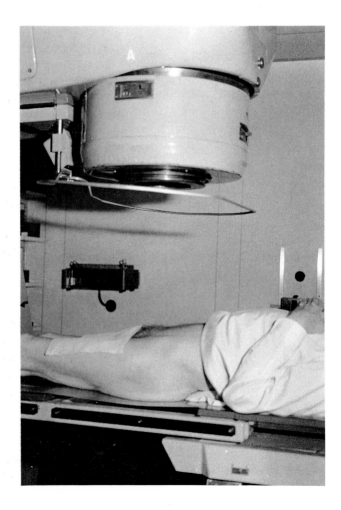

Fig. 15.6 Patient undergoing supervoltage radiotherapy with the linear accelerator.

Total cystectomy

Psychological preparations

Patients vary in their attitude towards cystectomy. Their age, relationships, feelings about their body and the distress caused by their symptoms all play a part. It is helpful to discuss the operation and its effects with the patient's partner as well as the patient. Booklets which explain the operation can be very useful because they stimulate appropriate questions, and allow the patient or their relatives to express their anxieties, which can then be explored.

General preparations

The patient needs to be fit enough to withstand a very severe operation. Anaemia, perhaps due to radiotherapy and haematuria, must be corrected by transfusion at least one week in advance. To prevent pulmonary complications, smoking ought to stop, and breathing exercises should be taught, along with leg exercises to prevent deep vein thrombosis.

The skin is shaved from nipples to knees, including the perineum.

Bowel preparation

The method of preparation of the bowel varies from one unit to another: to some extent they depend upon whether small or large bowel is to be used for the conduit, and upon the preference of the surgeon. In our unit we give a low residue diet supplemented by high protein drinks for 48 hours before operation, aperients are given until there is diarrhoea and at least 3 litres of clear fluid are given by mouth.

Selecting the site for the stoma

Placing the stoma in the right place is vitally important. The stoma should be put in an area of the abdomen free from creases when the patient sits, stands or bends. It must lie well away from the umbilicus, previous scars, the line of the belt, and hairy areas (Fig. 15.7) and it must be visible to the patient. Meeting all these requirements is not always easy.

Applicances

Today one can choose from a wide variety of drainable appliances with 'add on' facilities for overnight drainage (Fig. 15.8). The patient should have the opportunity to see and handle them, and make his or her choice in discussion with the nursing team. There are bags that can be used again or thrown away; disposable appliances supplied in one or in several pieces. Improvements are continually being made and alternative appliances can always be tried later. Eyesight, manual dexterity, life-style and the feeling

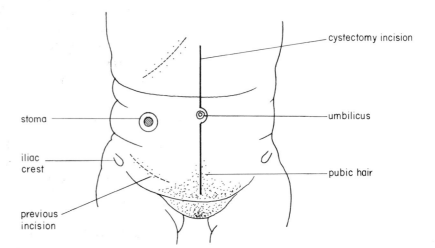

Fig. 15.7 The urinary stoma should be within easy reach of the patient, away from the umbilicus, previous scars, the pubic hair, and the line of the belt.

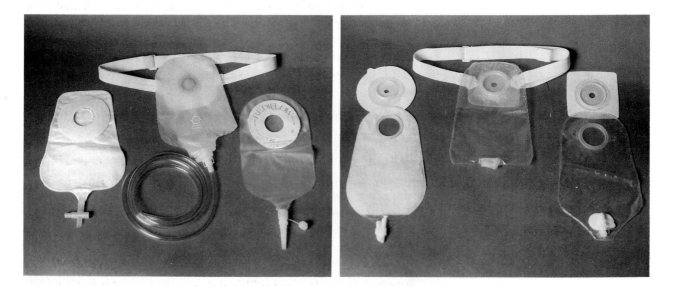

Fig. 15.8 There are many urinary stoma appliances to choose from.

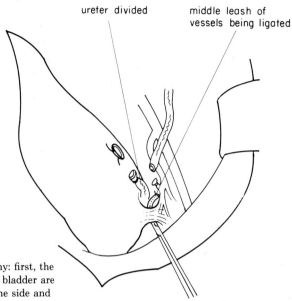

Fig. 15.9 Total cystectomy: first, the main vessels supplying the bladder are ligated and divided, first one side and then the other.

of security must all be thought of. Some men find it better to use braces rather than a belt. Women who normally wear a support belt may need to have it adjusted but usually there is no need to make any change in clothing.

For the patient who is a keen golfer the surgeon will try to fashion the stoma where it will not interfere with his swing. Another, in a wheel-chair, needs a stoma that is placed where the patient and his attendant can easily get at it. For all patients, who are starting a new life with a stoma, time spent choosing the position of the stoma and the appliance to go with it is time well spent.

The operation

Cystectomy needs a long incision. The main blood vessels to the bladder from the internal iliac artery are divided one after the other (Fig. 15.9). The urethra is cut across below the prostate except where there are multifocal tumours when the urethra is removed as well through an inconspicuous incision in the perineum.

When the bladder has been taken out there is a defect into which hang two severed ureters. Usually they are implanted into an *ileal conduit* made by isolating a loop of small intestine (Fig. 15.10). The ureters are joined to each other, splinted with 8 Ch nasogastric tubes, and then one end is

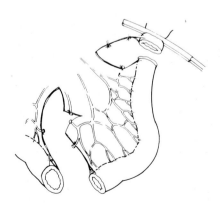

Fig. 15.10 An isolated loop of ileum is prepared for use as a urinary conduit.

sewn onto the loop of the bowel (Fig. 15.11) while the other end is brought to the skin as a *cutaneous urinary ileostomy or ileal conduit* (Fig. 15.12).

The urinary appliance must be applied carefully in the operating theatre. The theatre team will often have been on their feet for 6 to 8 hours after one of these operations and it is easy for them to hurry this last but crucial stage. Early leakage can be very demoralizing for the patient.

After the operation the bowel needs a period of rest, when there is a danger that the intestine will become distended. To keep the patient comfortable during this period of postoperative paralytic ileus a small *gastrostomy* (Fig. 15.13) tube is often placed in the stomach in preference to a nasogastric tube because it is more comfortable, can be left on free dependent drainage, and allows the patient to take some clear fluid by mouth as well as breathe and cough more easily.

Postoperative care

These patients lose a lot of fluid and blood during the operation and this *fluid must be replaced* accurately to maintain good hydration; this may need central and peripheral intravenous lines. The blood pressure and pulse will be carefully monitored in the early postoperative period, and the *urine output* is maintained at at least 30 ml/hr.

Enough *analgesia* must be given so as to allow the patient to breathe deeply and move in bed without pain. He can usually get up the day after operation. Narcotics may be required for several days to ensure relief of pain as well as provide adequate sleep.

The *gastrostomy* tube is clamped off when the patient has had a bowel

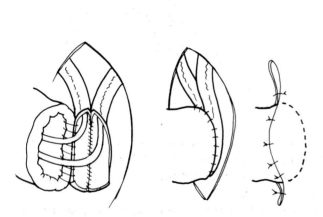

Fig. 15.11 The free ends of the ureters are joined to one end of the ileal conduit.

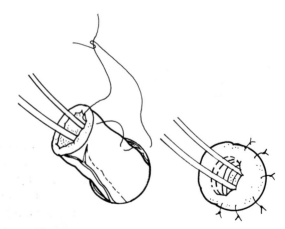

Fig. 15.12 The other end of the ileal conduit is brought out at the site previously marked.

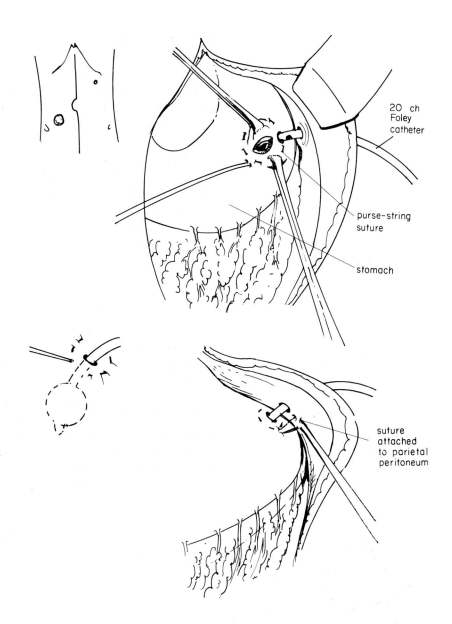

20 ch Foley catheter

purse-string suture

stomach

suture attached to parietal peritoneum

Fig. 15.13 A small gastrostomy tube in the stomach avoids the discomfort and irritation of a nasogastric tube.

action — 5 to 8 days after operation. It is removed after about 10 days. The gastrostomy is a simple Foley catheter. The balloon is let down and the retaining suture is cut. The hole between the stomach and the abdominal wall closes within a day or two.

When bowel sounds return there may be some diarrhoea. Reassure the patient that this is quite normal and will settle without any medication. A light diet can now be started, and increased as the appetite returns.

Low-dose *heparin* may be prescribed in addition to leg exercises to prevent deep vein thrombosis which is so common after operations in the pelvis. Appropriate antibiotics are always given because the urine is frequently infected in patients with bladder cancer.

The *drains* left in the pelvis are removed after 5 or 6 days. There is often some serous discharge from the perineum or penis especially when the patient stands up but excessive clear drainage, especially when associated with prolonged ileus, may mean a leak of urine and when in any doubt the creatinine content of this fluid should be measured. Loss of pus or faeces means the intestinal anastomosis has broken down — a rare complication but one that is more likely to occur after previous radiotherapy.

The *ureteric splints* will drain into the collecting appliance which is made of clear plastic so that one can check that the colour of the *stoma* is pink. At first the collecting appliance is connected to a bedside drainage bag, but when the patient starts to get up, he can set off on the road to independence by disconnecting, emptying and reconnecting the bag himself.

The *stoma bag* will first be changed after 4 or 5 days. At this time your patient will be watching your reaction. Encourage him to look at the stoma, and whenever possible, invite him to help get the new appliance ready. The stoma should always look pink and healthy, although there is always some oedema and mucus discharge. In these early days if a two-piece system is being used, it is less painful to apply it ready assembled.

Ureteric splints are removed after about 10 days and the patient can now apply the bags; he will need guidance and supervision. It will usually be necessary to change the bag only every 4 or 5 days but while he is learning to achieve his independence, a 'teaching session' may be needed more frequently. All the necessary equipment must be ready at hand, with the patient lying or standing in a convenient position where he can easily see the stoma.

As a high fluid intake is advised to prevent stasis of urine, it is a good idea to change the bag early in the morning, and never just after taking a diuretic when there is no controlling the flow. The surrounding skin must be dry or the appliance will not stick on; it may be removed before a warm but not a really hot bath for sweat will stop the new bag from sticking. Talcum powder too should only be used once the bag is securely in position. Supervision is needed until the patient feels confident, and encouragement and praise at their achievement will speed the process.

Before discharge, and with the patient's agreement, the person who will be looking after the patient at home should be involved in changing the bag. Warn them that the patient will be anxiously watching their reaction to the stoma. Now is the time to air worries and problems: this will avoid much of the apprehension and depression which is so often felt after leaving hospital.

It may be several weeks before the patient feels able to return to work. He should try to do a little more each day, and take up his hobbies as soon as possible. Most patients can return to work about 6 weeks after going home.

He will need a *supply of appliances* when he leaves hospital, together with a list of their order numbers. In Britain further appliances can be obtained on prescription but it is necessary that the general practitioner should be told roughly how many are likely to be needed every month.

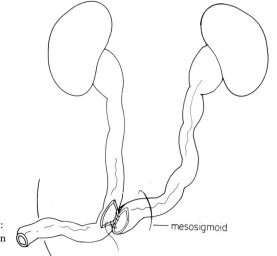

Fig. 15.14 Y-ureterostomy: a method of urinary diversion for ureters which are very dilated.

Visits from the community nurse and stoma therapist may also be arranged and most patients will benefit from joining the local branch of the Urinary Conduit Association, and their address and telephone number should be supplied.

Ureterostomy

This is a less traumatic form of urinary diversion which can be used when the ureters are obstructed and dilated. One ureter is joined to the other, in the form of a Y, and the longer one brought out on the skin as for an ileal conduit (Fig. 15.14). The blood supply of the ureter is much more precarious than that of the bowel, and there is a tendency for the end of the ureter to die back and lead to obstruction.

Sometimes ureterostomy is performed when it is found that the bladder cannot be removed but is giving rise to such severe symptoms that some form of palliative urinary diversion is needed. Before making the decision to offer this diversion, very careful consideration needs to be given to the provision of family support and future care.

Complications

The main early complications after cystectomy are infection in the wound and the chest, intestinal obstruction from adhesions and leakage from the anastomoses in the bowel and the ureters, causing prolonged ileus. Late complications are mainly concerned with the urinary stoma, hence the importance of making sure that the stoma is placed in the right position.

Continent diversions

When no radiotherapy has been used before the cystectomy it is possible to make use of the small or large intestine to fashion a continent urinary diversion in certain carefully selected cases (see p. 149).

Further reading

Breckman, B. (1981) *Stoma Care.* Beaconsfield Publishing, Beaconsfield.

Blandy, J. P. (1986) *Operative Urology*, 2nd edn. Blackwell Scientific Publications, Oxford.

Blandy, J. P., England, H. R., Evans, S. J. W., Hope-Stone, H. F., Mair, G. M. M., Mantell, B. S., Oliver, R. T. D., Paris, A. M. I. & Risdon, R. A. (1980) T3 bladder cancer — the case for salvage cystectomy. *British Journal of Urology*, **52**, 506–510.

Blandy, J. P., Tiptaft, R. C., Paris, A. M. I., Oliver, R. T. D. & Hope-Stone, H. F. (1985) The case for definitive radiotherapy and salvage cystectomy in localized bladder carcinoma. *World Journal of Urology*, **3**, 94–97.

Droller, M. J. (1985) Immunotherapy in genitourinary neoplasia. *Journal of Urology*, **133**, 1–5.

Fowler, C. G., Badenoch, D. F. & Thakar, D. R. (1984) Practical experience with flexible fibrescope cystoscopy in outpatients. *British Journal of Urology*, **56**, 618–621.

Health and Safety Executive (1983) *Precautions for the Safe Handling of Cytotoxic Drugs.* Guidance note ms 21. HSE, London. (The basic guidelines on handling cytotoxic drugs.)

Herr, H. W., Yagoda, A., Batata, M., Sogani, P. C. & Whitmore, W. F. (1983) Planned preoperative cisplatin and radiation therapy for locally advanced bladder cancer. *Cancer*, **52**, 2205–2208.

Moffatt, P. (1985) A revolution in urology (flexible fibreoptic cystoscopy). *Nursing Times*, 16 Oct., 30–31.

16 *Catheters and catheterization*

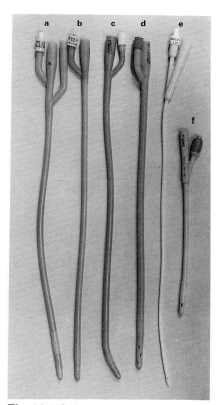

Fig. 16.1 Some of the varieties of urethral catheters in common use today: (a) three-way Foley irrigating, (b) two-way Foley, (c) Roberts' catheter with eye below balloon, (d) haematuria catheter with additional holes, (e) silicone elastomer catheter for long-term use, and (f) short female silicone elastomer catheter.

Fig. 16.2 Cross-section through three catheters showing the variation in the shape of the separate channels for irrigation and inflation.

Catheters

The catheter is the most important tool used by urologist and urological nurse. Its purpose is always the same — to let urine out of the collecting system. Catheters come in many different shapes and sizes, each designed for a particular situation.

Catheters have been known since the days of the Pharoahs of ancient Egypt, and down the centuries they have been made of many materials — silver, bronze, bamboo, silk stiffened with glue (gum-elastic) and innumerable varieties of rubber (Fig. 16.1). Today they are made from latex, polyvinyl choride, or silicone rubber. Of these, silicone rubber is the least irritating to the tissues and least likely to attract the deposition of calcium salts, but it is also the most expensive.

Catheters are never exactly circular in cross-section; some are more or less oval while others have ridges for the irrigating and inflating channels (Fig. 16.2) but then the urethra is never exactly circular in cross-section in either sex. When empty it is like an empty sock — when distended it is more or less oval, and in the male is ridged like the barrel of a rifle in the bulb. In the male the urethra is capable of considerable elongation during erection.

When filled out there is a limit to the size of the urethra, a limit that depends upon its circumference rather than its diameter. In most adult males, the maximum circumference of the urethra is about 25 mm. This is useful because instruments are seldom circular in cross-section.

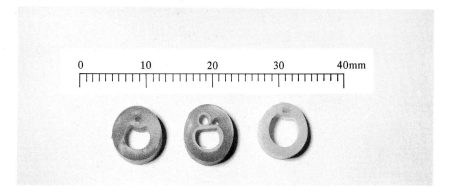

0 10 20 30 40mm

Size of catheters

Catheters are graded according to their circumference in millimetres. This scale was devised by Charrière, a French instrument maker when the metric system was first introduced after the French revolution and it is referred to as the Charrière (Ch) or French (F) scale. (There is another system sometimes used for smaller catheters, named after Béniqué (Bé) which is calibrated in half-millimetres.)

Clear urine without clots or debris will flow easily down a 12 Ch or 14 Ch urethral catheter. If you cut across a modern catheter you will find considerable differences in the size of the channel for urine. Much of the inside of a catheter may be taken up by channels for inflating the balloon or for irrigation. The more of these additional channels, the less room for the urine to escape.

Choice of catheter

When the only purpose of the catheter is to let out clear urine it needs only to be a thin, soft tube which is removed as soon as the bladder is emptied out. More often it is necessary to keep the catheter in the bladder and for this purpose the Foley catheter was designed with a balloon to stop it slipping out. The inflatable balloon should be filled with the least amount of fluid that will stop it falling out of the bladder. A shorter catheter may be used for women.

If a catheter is so big that it fits the urethra tightly it will block the paraurethral ducts and bacteria will breed inside them to form *paraurethral abscesses*. If these heal it is with scar tissue that will contract and narrow the urethra but they may burst outside the urethra and allow urine to escape into the tissues or work its way through the skin as a urinary fistula (Figs. 16.3 and 16.4).

Too large a catheter may also lead to blockage and infection of the ejaculatory ducts which is followed by *epididymitis*, or of the prostatic ducts causing *prostatitis* or a *prostatic abscess* (Fig. 16.5).

Where the catheter lies up against the urethra wall, it can give rise to a pressure sore which in time heals with scar tissue which will contract and cause a stricture of the urethra. These pressure sores tend to be seen at the level of the external sphincter, the external urinary meatus and where the urethra is angulated at the junction of penis and scrotum (Fig. 16.6).

The lesson is clear; use only the smallest catheter that is needed to let out the urine and which will allow plenty of room between catheter and urethra for the secretions of the paraurethral and prostatic glands to escape (Fig. 16.7).

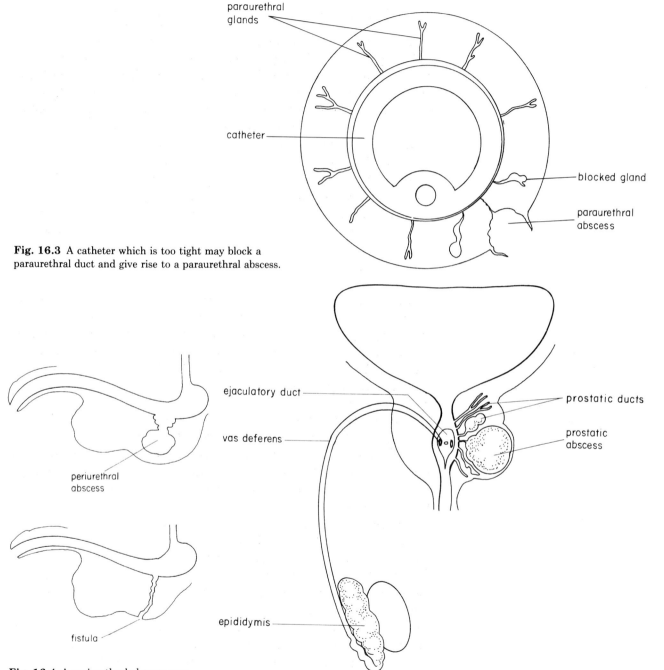

Fig. 16.3 A catheter which is too tight may block a paraurethral duct and give rise to a paraurethral abscess.

Fig. 16.4 A periurethral abscess may burst into the subcutaneous tissues of the scrotum, and if it ruptures through the skin, become a urethral fistula.

Fig. 16.5 A catheter which is too tight may block the prostatic and ejaculatory ducts leading to a prostatic abscess and epididymitis.

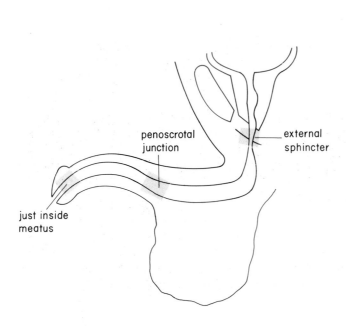

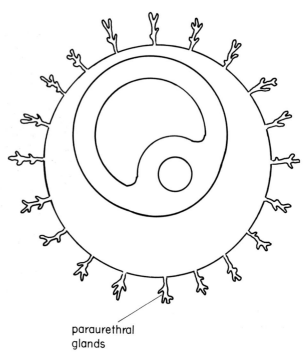

penoscrotal
junction

external
sphincter

just inside
meatus

paraurethral
glands

Fig. 16.6 Pressure sores may form where the catheter presses against the urethra near the meatus, at the penoscrotal angle, and near the external sphincter.

Fig. 16.7 A catheter should be small enough to allow the secretions of the paraurethral ducts to escape easily.

Catheterization

Explain the procedure to the patient. Make sure that his or her privacy is ensured, and protect the bed by a waterproof sheet under the buttocks. Good light is always needed especially when women are to be catheterized, and without an assistant it can be difficult to preserve aseptic technique and prevent undue exposure of the patient.

Equipment

The following equipment should be available on a cleaned trolley (Fig. 16.8):
two catheters of an appropriate size and type;
sterile drapes;
sterile wool swabs and forceps;
antiseptic in sterile containers;
sterile lubricant and nozzle (1% lignocaine with 0.25% chlorhexidine);
specimen container;
sterile drainage bag and clean holder and stand;
sterile syringe with 5–30 ml sterile water;

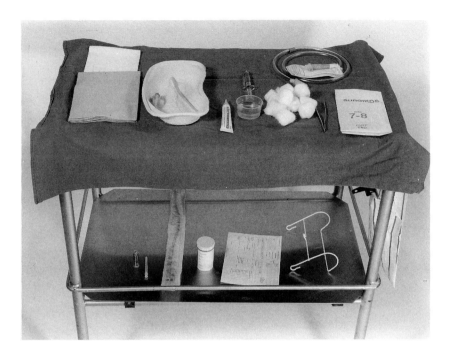

Fig. 16.8 Equipment needed for catheterization.

sterile gloves of appropriate size;
sterile gauze swabs;
a penile clamp for male catheterization.

Catheterization in the female

The patient lies comfortably on her back with her legs flexed and rotated outwards (Fig. 16.9). Drape sterile towels over the abdomen and legs to form a sterile field on the bed between the legs.

Wearing gloves, and working from the right side of the bed, with the equipment within easy reach of your right hand, use your left thumb and forefinger to separate the labia and hold them apart (Fig. 16.10). (This is reversed for left-handed operators.)

Holding swabs in forceps, dip them in antiseptic solution and swab the perineal area towards the rectum using each swab only once.

Identify the urethra and vagina and instil about 5 ml of the antiseptic-anaesthetic gel into the urethra. Leave it for a minute.

Keeping the end of the catheter in the receiver, which is placed on the bed between the patient's legs, gently pass the tip into the urethra for 6 to 7 cm until the urine flows.

If the catheter is to remain in place fill its balloon using the syringe of

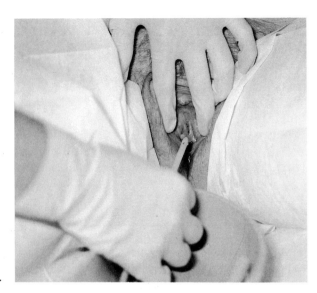

Fig. 16.9 A female patient in the position ready for catheterization.

sterile water and gently draw it down to make sure that it is secure. Connect the tubing of the drainage bag and secure it to the thigh to prevent it from being dislodged as she moves around (Fig. 16.11).

If the catheter is to be removed, let all the urine flow out and press gently on the suprapubic area and ask the patient to cough as you withdraw the catheter. Measure the volume of urine that has been withdrawn. When necessary send a sample to the laboratory in a sterile pot for bacteriological culture.

Catheterization in the male

The patient lies comfortably, and the whole penis is cleaned with antiseptic, paying special attention to the glans and its meatus. Place a waterproof drape with a hole in it over the penis to provide a sterile field. Inject 15 ml of 1% lignocaine-chlorhexidine gel slowly into the meatus, (Fig. 16.12) and milk it down the urethra. Apply a penile clamp transversely across the urethra to keep in the gel. It needs 5 minutes for effective anaesthesia (Fig. 16.13).

Hold the penis in the left hand almost at right angles to the body, and pass the tip of the catheter gently down the urethra. A little resistance will be felt when the catheter reaches the external sphincter; ask the patient to try to pass water — this allows the sphincter to relax and the catheter will then slip through.

If any difficulty is encountered, medical staff should be called. Never use any force. The lining of the urethra is very thin and easily torn.

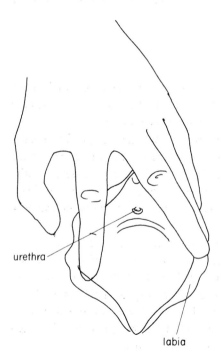

Fig. 16.10 Separate the labia with the fingers of the left hand.

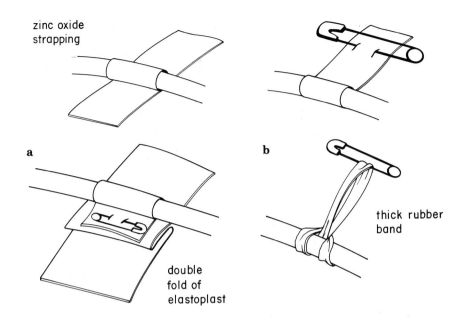

zinc oxide strapping

double fold of elastoplast

a

b

thick rubber band

Fig. 16.11 The drainage tubing is secured to the thigh to prevent it being dislodged as the patient walks about (a), or pinned to bedlinen or clothing to prevent dragging on tubing (b).

Fig. 16.12 Catheterization of a male: instilling local anaesthetic — antiseptic gel.

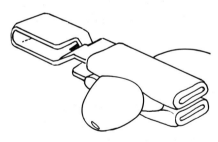

Fig. 16.13 The local anaesthetic is retained for 5 minutes with a penile clamp.

Suprapubic catheterization

When it is not possible to pass a urethral catheter on a patient with acute retention of urine it will be necessary for medical staff to insert a catheter suprapubically. In such a patient the bladder is easily felt.

The pubic hair is shaved and the area cleansed. Using a fine needle about 0.5 ml of 1% lignocaine is injected into the dermis to raise a weal about 2 cm above the symphysis pubis (Fig. 16.14). Using a longer needle, more local anaesthetic is injected through the weal towards the bladder, until urine is aspirated. An artery forceps placed on the needle marks how far the bladder is below the skin (Fig. 16.15).

With a no. 10 blade a nick is made in the skin about 4 mm long and the special suprapubic catheter which fits over a sharp trochar is pushed firmly into the bladder for 2 or 3 cm longer than the distance measured on the needle (Fig. 16.16). The trochar is withdrawn and the rest of the catheter is advanced into the bladder being held firmly so that it cannot fall out as the bladder is emptied. Connect the catheter to the drainage tube and bag as soon as possible.

Some of these cannulae have balloons to keep them in the bladder and others have retaining collars that are sutured to the skin (Fig. 16.17). A

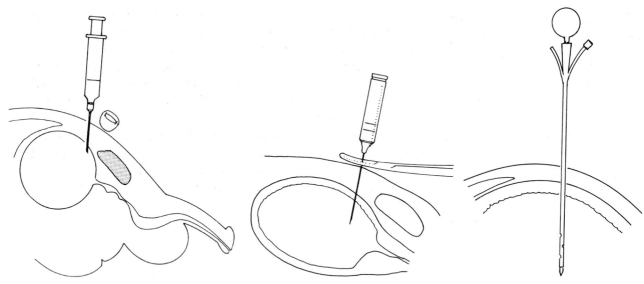

Fig. 16.14 Suprapubic cystostomy: local anaesthetic is injected as far as the bladder until urine is aspirated.

Fig. 16.15 An artery forceps is placed on the needle to mark the distance between bladder and skin.

Fig. 16.16 The trochar and cannula are advanced into the bladder.

dressing is applied around the site, and the catheter and tube are secured with adhesive to the skin so that they cannot be accidentally dislodged when the patient moves around.

Intermittent self-catheterization

There are many reasons, especially in neuropathic disorders of the bladder, when patients cannot empty the bladder. A permanent indwelling catheter can be avoided if they can learn how to pass a catheter for themselves several times a day. Although strict aseptic technique is essential in hospital to prevent cross infection, a 'clean' technique at home when it is done only by the patient, carries less risk of infection than an indwelling catheter. The patient needs to be able to reach the area with both hands to manipulate the catheter, and must be motivated, encouraged, and helped to persevere until he or she is confident.

For the *male* patient, it is a relatively easy technique, as the meatus can easily be seen and the catheter inserted.

For the *female* patient, a little lesson in anatomy may be needed. Let her lie on a couch, with a good light directed at the perineum. Show her her urethra with the aid of a mirror (Fig. 16.18). Let her palpate the urethra using the middle finger of her left hand, while the index and ring finger are used to separate the labia (Fig. 16.19). A 12 Ch Jaques catheter

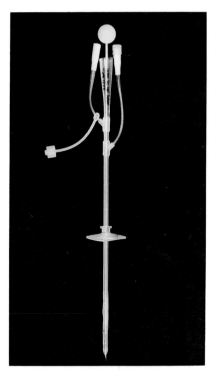

is dipped into lubricant, passed into the urethra (Fig. 16.20) and left in position until the urine stops flowing. It is generally a mixture of amazement and delight that greets the first successful attempt.

If she is unsteady on her feet or generally rather frail your patient may need to pass the catheter lying down, first making sure that the bed or couch is protected, and that the end of the catheter can drain into a suitable large clean receptacle.

Most patients find it best to use the toilet where some prefer to sit and others raise one leg onto the side of the lavatory pan or a low stool, and direct the flow of urine from the catheter into the pan.

While learning in hospital, a sterile catheter is used each time, but at

Fig. 16.17 Several different kinds of disposable suprapubic cannulae are available: some have a self-retaining balloon, others have to be sutured to the skin to keep them in position.

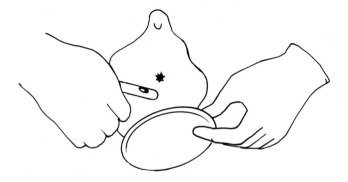

Fig. 16.18 A mirror helps to show a female where the urethra is situated.

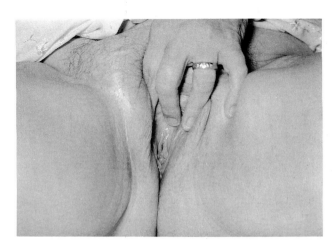

Fig. 16.19 Her index and ring fingers separate her labia, while she feels for the urethra with the middle finger.

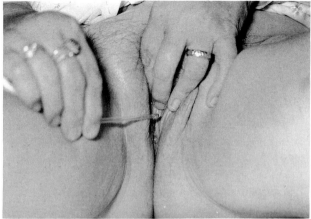

Fig. 16.20 Self-catheterization using the toilet: some prefer to sit, others raise one leg on the side of the pan.

home the catheters can be rinsed, washed, dried and used again for a week before being discarded. In Britain appropriate catheters are available on a doctor's prescription. Short ones are available for women.

It is important to stress the need to keep the bladder regularly and completely emptied out. How often the catheter should be passed will depend on how much urine is produced and so the patient should check this from time to time, and make sure the volume is kept below 500 ml. Most patients quickly learn to pass their catheters in the lavatory, and their life-style is enhanced rather than inhibited in any way.

Indwelling catheter

As catheterization and catheter drainage always carry a risk of infection catheters should never be left indwelling unless really necessary. They are often required for retention of urine, or after surgery.

How can we reduce the risk of infection?

1 *Ensure an aseptic technique* when passing the catheter.

2 *Make sure that the catheter is secure*, able to drain freely, and not likely to become twisted, kinked or disconnected.

3 *Never clamp off a catheter* without specific instructions. Clamping may be needed when there is another outlet for urine e.g. a nephrostomy or a suprapubic catheter, or when cytotoxic drugs are being instilled into the bladder.

4 *Never spigot a catheter.* The old idea of 'training the bladder' or 'regaining tone' is nonsense, for example, bladders kept empty for many years quickly recover normal function once a renal transplant starts to make urine.

5 *Keep drainage bags below the level of the bladder* on the correct stands or holders; urine will not run uphill, and failure to do this is as bad as clamping off the catheter.

6 *Ensure a high fluid intake whenever possible.* There may be rare exceptions, e.g. in renal failure, when intake is restricted.

7 *Never use a catheter that is larger than necessary.*

8 *Use drainage bags* which are part of a closed system and with a non-return valve, emptying tap, and sampling port for short-term use (Fig. 16.21). For longer-term use, 'leg' or 'porta' bags may be worn under the clothing but they must have adequate capacity for the day. At night a larger bag is added on to give additional capacity. It is wasteful, and potentially dangerous, to change bags night and morning.

9 *Spread catheterized patients round the ward* rather than having them in adjacent beds to prevent cross infection. Empty their bags when other attention is given rather than on a 'round'. Use clean, sterilized jugs.

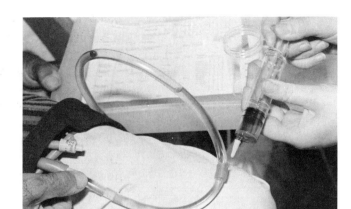

Fig. 16.21 A sampling port with a rubber sleeve allows samples of urine to be obtained with a needle from the drainage tubing.

10 *Always wash your hands and dry them carefully* when emptying bags and disposing of urine.

11 *Never disconnect a catheter bag without good reason.* Bags can safely be left for a week if intact. If bags must be changed, use a strict aseptic technique, and carefully clean the connection with antiseptic.

12 *Only irrigate the bladder when it is essential*: 'milking' a catheter will often relieve a slight blockage more safely.

13 *Keep the area round the catheter insertion clean and free from encrustation* preferably with soap and water once or twice a day. There is no reason why a patient should not take a shower or a bath, if his general condition otherwise allows, but the drainage system must be kept intact.

14 *Provide clean dressings* around suprapubic and nephrostomy tubes. Report any infection or leakage.

15 *Monitor infection* by regular bacteriological examination.

16 *Avoid antibiotics* if the patient is well and not otherwise at risk, to prevent the development of resistant organisms.

17 *Always replace the foreskin in an uncircumcised male* after performing catheter toilet to prevent *paraphimosis* (see p. 211).

Changing a catheter

Indwelling catheters must be changed before they are blocked off to prevent the dangerous time-bomb of having infected urine under pressure inside the bladder. The time it takes for calcium salts to block a catheter can very considerably from one patient to another. This clogging process is more rapid when there is infection with a urea-splitting organism such as *Proteus mirabilis*, and can be slowed down if the patient drinks enough to keep the urine well diluted.

When the catheter is changed the balloon is let down by aspirating the sterile water. There is often a thin crust of calcium salts on the surface of the balloon which will crack off as the balloon is let down (Fig. 16.22) leaving particles in the bladder that will act as the nucleus for a stone to form. After changing the catheter the bladder should be gently irrigated several times with a bladder syringe and sterile water (Fig. 16.23) to remove these particles of crust.

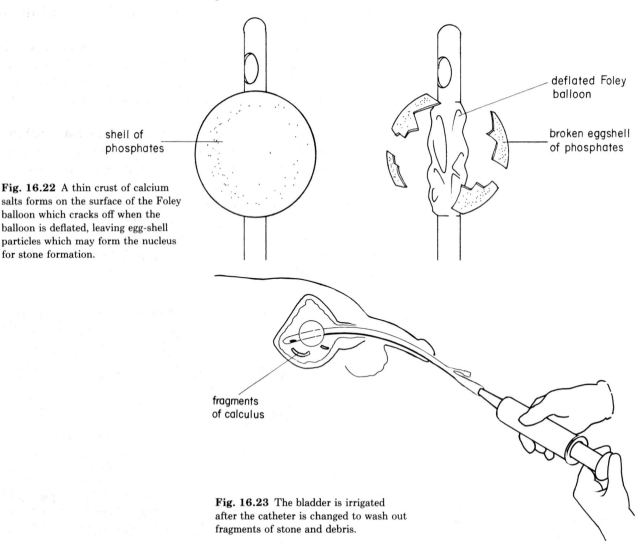

shell of
phosphates

deflated Foley
balloon

broken eggshell
of phosphates

Fig. 16.22 A thin crust of calcium salts forms on the surface of the Foley balloon which cracks off when the balloon is deflated, leaving egg-shell particles which may form the nucleus for stone formation.

fragments
of calculus

Fig. 16.23 The bladder is irrigated after the catheter is changed to wash out fragments of stone and debris.

When the Foley balloon will not go down

Every now and again the self-retaining balloon of a Foley catheter fails to deflate. There are several ways of dealing with this, and the anxious patient may be assured that the catheter will be removed. Medical staff are informed. Whatever you do *never inject ether down the channel* to rupture the balloon. Deaths have occurred from this practice; vaporization of the ether may so expand the balloon as to rupture the bladder and the ether itself may damage the wall of the bladder. Stones may form on the fragments left behind.

Proceed in the following steps:

1 Inject 1–2 ml of water or air up the balloon channel, and try to withdraw the water.

2 Cut off the balloon channel at its junction with the main stem of the catheter (Fig. 16.24); the fluid will then often ooze out slowly. Unless there is some pressing medical reason to remove the catheter at once, leave it to empty slowly over the next 24 hours, and the catheter will fall out of its own accord.

3 If it is urgently necessary to remove the catheter a fine ureteric catheter with its stillette (Fig. 16.25) is lubricated, and passed up the balloon channel; if the water does not run out when the stillette is removed, try pushing it in again to prick the balloon.

4 If none of these methods succeed the catheter is gently pulled down until its balloon can be felt in the perineum, where after injecting a little local anaesthetic a fine needle is inserted to prick the balloon (Fig. 16.26). An alternative method is to locate the balloon with ultrasound and pass the needle suprapubically (Fig. 16.27).

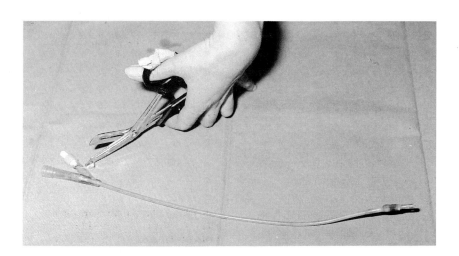

Fig. 16.24 If the channel for the Foley balloon is cut off, the fluid may run out slowly over the next hour or two.

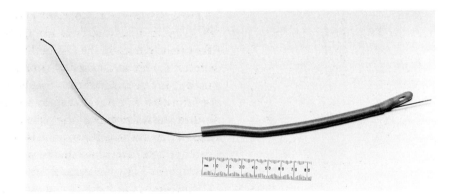

Fig. 16.25 A fine ureteric catheter with a wire stylette is lubricated and passed up the balloon channel.

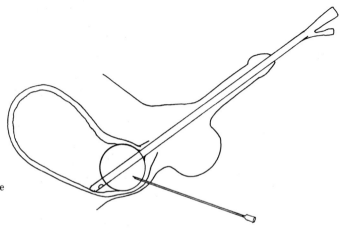

Fig. 16.26 If the catheter is drawn down firmly until the balloon is felt on the perineum, it can be ruptured with a fine needle.

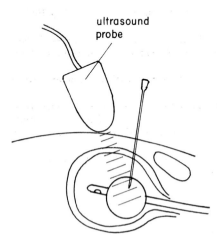

ultrasound probe

Fig. 16.27 The balloon may be ruptured with a fine needle introduced through the bladder under ultrasound control.

The 'leaking' catheter

Urine may leak around the catheter for a number of reasons. Follow this check-list:

1 *Is the drainage bag below the level of the bladder?*

2 *Is the tubing kinked?*

3 *Is the catheter blocked.* The cause of the block may be blood clot, pus, stones or a chip of prostate. If 'milking' the catheter does not clear the obstruction, it may be necessary to irrigate or change the catheter. After surgery or trauma analgesia should only be used as a stop gap while medical staff tackle the underlying problem. Nurses should not attempt to remove or replace catheters in these situations because it is so easy to add to the damage.

4 *Is the patient having bladder spasms?* Especially after operations in the region of the trigone the detrusor is very apt to contract. The patient will feel pain and an intense desire to pass urine. The catheter will be draining freely, but during the spasm more urine will leak around the

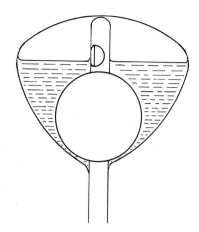

Fig. 16.28 In most catheters the drainage holes are above the balloon.

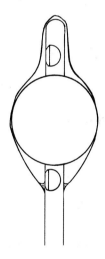

Fig. 16.29 In a Roberts catheter there is a drainage hole downstream of the balloon.

catheter. Of course the patient may well not understand how a catheter works or that such spasms are quite innocent and an explanation will often relieve his fear that something has gone wrong. Antispasmodics or sedatives such as diclofenac, propantheline or diazepam may give relief but if, for example, after radiotherapy, the spasms become intolerable they may have to be relieved by a caudal epidural anaesthetic.

5 *How much water is in the balloon*? The more water in the balloon, the larger it is, and the higher it lies in the bladder. In most catheters the drainage holes are above the balloon (Fig. 16.28) and if urine accumulates below the balloon it may leak around the catheter. The less fluid in the balloon, the smaller will be this space for the urine to collect in. If a larger balloon is needed a Roberts catheter (Fig. 16.29) may be used, which has an extra eye downstream of the balloon.

6 *How long has the indwelling catheter been in position*? The urethra and sphincter may lose their tone when a catheter has been in position for many months. It seldom helps to replace the catheter with a larger one; the reverse is more likely to be the case, and a smaller catheter may not leak.

7 *How large a balloon can the patient push out*? After many weeks almost every measure seems to fail and patients expel catheters even when the balloon has been filled with 40 ml of water. The time has then come to consider the question of urinary diversion (see p. 147).

Further reading

Belfield, P. W., Young, J. B. & Mulley, G. P. (1985) Rejection of catheters. *British Medical Journal*, **291**, 108–109.

Blandy, J. P. (1986) *Operative Urology*, 2nd edn. Blackwell Scientific Publications, Oxford.

Browning, G. G. P., Barr, L. & Horsburgh, A. G. (1984) Management of obstructed balloon catheters. *British Medical Journal*, **289**, 89–91.

McCabe, S. E. & Paterson, J. G. (1984) Management of obstructed balloon catheters. *British Medical Journal*, **289**, 837.

Meers, P. D., Cartwright, R. Y., Mayon-White, R., Clifford, C., Webster, M. & Jenner, E. A. (1982) Urinary tract infection; the role of the nurse. *Proceedings of Conference Organized by Nursing Practice Research Unit at Northwick Park Hospital and Clinical Research Centre.* DHSS, London.

Reynolds, M.A. (1982) *Clean Intermittent Catheterization: CURN Project.* Michigan Nurses' Association. Grune & Stratton, New York

17 *The prostate*

Anatomy

Imagine the prostate as a pair of croissants, one above the other, thin in front, and thick behind. These are the two *zones* of the prostate. The urethra passes through the middle of them, and the ejaculatory ducts enter the back of the urethra in the gap between the upper and lower zones to open on a little bump — the *verumontanum* (Fig. 17.1). Each zone of the prostate is made up of little glands rather like toothpaste tubes each provided with a sleeve of muscle to squeeze it out into the urethra. We have little idea of the purpose of these glands, except that they add a small amount to the seminal fluid.

There are two important rings of muscle which run among the glands that make up the prostate (Fig. 17.2) the *internal sphincter* or *bladder neck* at its upper end, and the *distal sphincter mechanism* at its lower end. This distal sphincter mechanism is actually made of two parts: one made of involuntary muscle which surrounds the urethra just below the verumontanum and just above the membranous urethra — the '*supra-membranous sphincter*' and is the really important part of the sphincter that is capable of sustained contraction. Below it lies a ring of voluntary muscle that is part of the levator ani, which can contract only for a short time (Fig. 17.3).

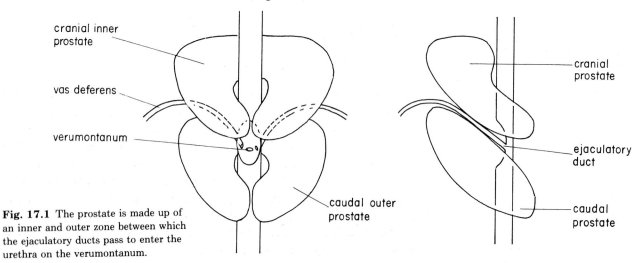

cranial inner prostate

vas deferens

verumontanum

cranial prostate

ejaculatory duct

caudal outer prostate

caudal prostate

Fig. 17.1 The prostate is made up of an inner and outer zone between which the ejaculatory ducts pass to enter the urethra on the verumontanum.

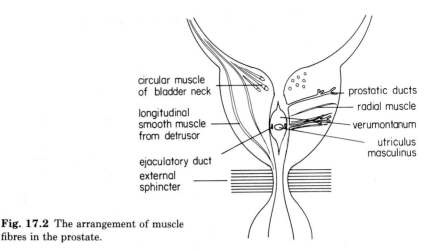

Fig. 17.2 The arrangement of muscle fibres in the prostate.

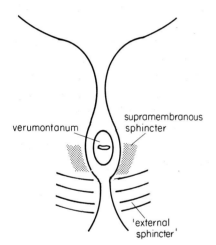

Fig. 17.3 The distal sphincter mechanism is made of two parts: the 'external' voluntary part and the 'supramembranous' involuntary part.

Arteries

The prostate has a rich arterial blood supply from branches of the internal iliac artery.

Veins and lymphatics

In addition to the expected set of veins and lymphatics draining into those of the pelvis, the prostate has extra private 'back-door' connections with the lymphatics and veins of the pelvis, the upper end of each femur and the lumbar vertebrae, so that cancer or microorganisms in the prostate easily spread to these bones.

Diseases of the prostate

Benign enlargement of the prostate

This is a process which affects the upper inner zone of the prostate and is found to some extent in every man after the age of 40. It is part of the normal ageing process; it cannot be prevented, and in 90% of men it does no harm. Benign enlargement consists of an increase in the bulk of the normal connective tissue, glands and muscle fibres of the inner zone of the prostate. It may make the gland more stiff and rigid, or it may form lumps which distort the gland and compress the urethra. These lumps are often mistakenly referred to as the 'lobes' of the prostate.

As these lumps enlarge they compress the outer and lower zone, flattening it into a so-called *'capsule'* (Fig. 17.4). The operation of

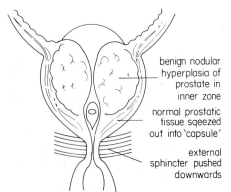

Fig. 17.4 In benign prostatic hypertrophy, nodules form in the inner zone which compress the remaining healthy tissue of the outer zone into a 'capsule'.

benign nodular hyperplasia of prostate in inner zone

normal prostatic tissue sqeezed out into 'capsule'

external sphincter pushed downwards

prostatectomy consists of the removal of this hypertrophied inner zone from within the capsule. It may be either an open operation, or a transurethral resection (Fig. 17.5).

Prostatic outflow obstruction

Either because of its stiffness or the bulk of the lumps of benign hypertrophy, the outflow of urine from the bladder is obstructed. This may occur to a slight extent in all men but in only about 10% is the obstruction severe enough to need an operation.

The bladder responds to the increased outflow resistance by hypertrophy of the detrusor muscle, whose fibres become coarser and change in texture from a fine felt to an open-woven network (*trabeculation*). As the pressure inside the bladder increases, so its lining of urothelium may balloon out through the gaps between the coarse fibres to form little pockets — *saccules and diverticula* (Fig. 17.6).

A little hypertrophy of the detrusor muscle causes no harm; the bladder still empties out completely, and although the patient may notice some increased frequency and a need to pass urine more urgently, because the hypertrophied detrusor is also more jumpy, there is no danger. But if the process continues the detrusor gets tired and begins to give up the struggle. Its muscle fibres stretch and can no longer contract effectively so the bladder begins to accumulate *residual urine* (Fig. 17.7). There is now a danger that this residual urine will become infected — the patient is carrying the urological time-bomb of infected urine under pressure.

If the process is allowed to continue unchecked, the increasing bulk of the prostate may lift up and kink the ureters where they enter the bladder causing them to become obstructed (Fig. 17.8) and now each kidney becomes hydronephrotic and loses tissue from the medulla, with the result that it can no longer process the glomerular filtrate, concentrate the urine, conserve salt or acidify the urine (see p. 30). Eventually the process of atrophy extends to the cortex of the kidney and there is a reduction in glomerular filtration; only at this late stage do the blood urea and creatinine begin to rise — *uraemia.*

At any time the kidney's rate of deterioration may be accelerated by infection, for if infected urine is forced into kidneys under pressure, inflammation increases the damage already caused by back-pressure (see p. 110).

Detrusor failure

This may be sudden or gradual. *Acute retention* of urine may occur without any warning in a patient with prostatic outflow obstruction;

transurethral prostatectomy

enucleative prostatectomy

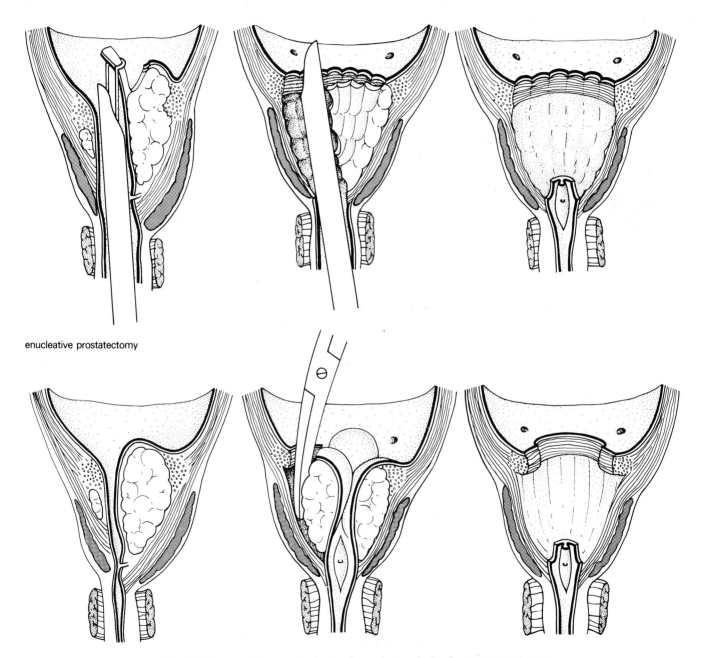

Fig. 17.5 In prostatectomy for benign hyperplasia, whether by open operation or transurethral resection, the inner zone with its nodules is removed from the compressed outer zone or capsule.

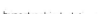
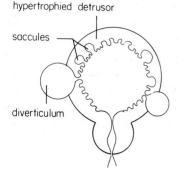

Fig. 17.6 With hypertrophy of the detrusor muscle its fibres become more coarse and gaps appear between them allowing the lining mucosa of the bladder to bulge out as saccules and diverticula.

sometimes after another illness or operation, sometimes when the patient allows the bladder to get overfull, and occasionally when he gets drunk. The bladder becomes full of urine under high pressure and is intensely painful.

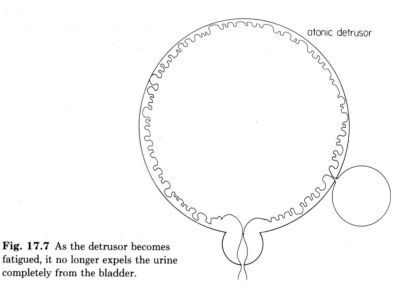

Fig. 17.7 As the detrusor becomes fatigued, it no longer expels the urine completely from the bladder.

Fig. 17.8 If obstruction is unrelieved and hypertrophy of the detrusor continues, eventually the ureters become obstructed.

Chronic retention by contrast occurs gradually and without pain. The volume of residual urine in the failing bladder gets larger and larger, the detrusor muscle fibres become more and more stretched, and the bladder enlarges and swells up in the abdomen like a pregnancy. After a time the stretched detrusor fibres begin to hold the neck of the bladder half-open, and urine runs away — *chronic retention with overflow.* By the time this happens there is usually enough damage to the renal tubules to cause dehydration and loss of salt, and enough loss of the cortex to give an elevated creatinine and urea.

Management of benign enlargement of the prostate

IN ACUTE RETENTION

The patient is admitted to hospital in pain and unable to pass urine. Other causes of acute retention of urine such as a spinal injury or acute neurological illness must be excluded by a careful examination but usually there is a long-standing history of previous prostatic outflow symptoms — hesitancy, poor stream, frequency, or getting up during the night to pass urine.

The patient in acute retention has severe pain, and needs a suitable dose of morphine for it. Sometimes with morphine and being put into a warm bath, he is able to pass water, and this should be the first line of treatment.

If he is unable to pass water in the bath, then a *catheter* is passed (see p. 186). If a small soft catheter does not enter the bladder easily, the house-surgeon may insert a *suprapubic cystostomy* tube (see p. 187). In some hospitals this is the preferred method of draining the bladder in acute retention. With both these methods the urine is collected by a closed drainage system to a bag, and the relief to the patient is instant and enormous. A small sample is sent to the laboratory for culture. In acute retention all the urine is let out of the bladder at once.

In a number of patients the episode of acute retention has been brought on by some other event, e.g. a chest infection, myocardial infarct, or a bout of constipation. In such patients once they have recovered from the precipitating illness or when, say, their bowel has been cleared, the catheter may be removed to see if they can empty their bladder — if necessary measuring the residual with ultrasound or a catheter to ensure that the bladder is being emptied completely. The usual patient with a long crescendo history of prostatic symptoms, provided he is otherwise fit, is then prepared for prostatectomy within the next few days.

CHRONIC RETENTION

The *nursing management* of these patients needs far more care. When the bladder is grossly enlarged and the patient is uraemic, the bladder is drained (as above) with a urethral or suprapubic catheter.

It is usual to let the urine out relatively slowly by placing a clamp on the tubing and allowing a specific volume (about 300 ml) to drain out each hour until the bladder is empty, and then continue free drainage. There are different views as to the need for this *slow decompression*. It may make for less bleeding when the pressure inside the bladder is let down, and it is usually prudent to make changes slowly in the volume of the body compartments in old people. However, the volume of urine coming out of the bladder must be carefully measured and recorded hour by hour, for when the pressure is relieved in the urinary tract, there is often a *post-obstructive diuresis.*

The renal tubules, working for such a long time against a raised pressure, find themselves coping with a huge volume of glomerular filtrate that now rushes past them. They cannot concentrate the urine or reabsorb salt. Very large volumes of urine are sometimes passed — up to 24 litres in 24 hours in one of our patients. This may give rise to such a severe shortage of extracellular and blood volume that the patient becomes shocked and may die.

These old men are already tired, dehydrated and uraemic and in addition often have urinary infections. They are often bewildered and frightened. Catheterization affords them much needed rest, because they do not need to make frequent trips to the toilet, but their general condition must be monitored carefully.

They must be weighed on admission, after the bladder has been emptied, and then daily at a regular time. Weight changes will reflect fluid changes. A strict fluid balance chart must also be kept.

During the early *diuretic phase* the blood pressure is recorded hourly to detect hypotension. Oral fluids are encouraged and salt supplements given by mouth. By these means it may be possible to keep pace with the diuresis, but when the patient is uraemic he is often so nauseated that he cannot drink enough or keep tablets down. He may need antiemetics. Not only will his dry mouth need care, but many litres of intravenous normal saline with added potassium chloride may be needed to replace lost fluid and salts and restore a normal balance. Serum electrolyte and urea levels are checked at least once a day during the diuretic phase. By these means the blood urea and creatinine fall once obstruction has been relieved and his dehydration has been corrected. When his appetite returns and he is able to eat, a special diet is usually not necessary.

Fortunately after a few days the tubules recover and large quantities of water and salt are no longer needed. But with rehydration another problem is uncovered — anaemia. Often these old men are very anaemic on admission, but it may not be obvious because they are so dehydrated that there is an abnormally small circulating blood volume. When their shortage of salt and water has been corrected, a repeat measurement of the haemoglobin may reveal a severe anaemia and several units of blood may be necessary before they are ready for an operation.

It is usual for a man in chronic retention to take 6 or 7 days to adjust his fluid balance, recover from post-obstructive diuresis, and receive a blood transfusion. When the daily record of his plasma creatinine shows that it has reached a steady plateau, lower than which it will not fall, then — and only then — is prostatectomy performed.

PROSTATECTOMY

The object of 'prostatectomy' is to remove the obstructing benign tissue from the inner zone leaving the compressed outer zone or 'capsule' behind, as well as the two components of the distal sphincter mechanism that lie downstream of the verumontanum — the supramembranous and external striated sphincter.

The 'adenoma' of the inner zone can be removed by transurethral resection or by an open operation (Fig. 17.5).

TRANSURETHRAL RESECTION OF THE PROSTATE — TURP

Preoperative care

A *urine* sample must be cultured so that correct antibiotics can be given if they are needed.

Not only will the patient be more comfortable after operation if he is not *constipated*, but a good bowel movement before prostatectomy will avoid straining after the operation which may cause bleeding.

He will need to be aware that he will be *catheterized* for at least 2 days after the operation, and that saline will be run in and out of the bladder. Explain that some bleeding is inevitable and that the *irrigation* is to prevent blood from clotting in the bladder. The catheter and operation should cause only mild discomfort, and any pain should be reported to the nursing staff so that it can be relieved.

Fluids will be given intravenously for the first few hours, but a little can be taken by mouth once the patient is fully recovered from the anaesthetic. He will be allowed to eat normally the next day.

As the *stay in hospital* is only 4 to 5 days, it is important to be sure that the patient has someone to look after him when he leaves. *Secondary haemorrhage* is always a possibility and to prevent this, the patient must avoid strenuous physical effort until the scab caused by the diathermy in the prostatic fossa has had time to separate — usually about 10 to 14 days. It is also important to keep the urine free from infection, and to treat any infection appropriately.

This needs to be spelt out to many men, especially doctors and self-employed business men; they must not go back to work, drive the car, dig the garden, play golf, or carry heavy shopping for the first two weeks. Most men are terrified of another 'stoppage' and can avoid this by resting, and drinking more than usual — especially at the first sign of bleeding.

Men undergoing prostatectomy should be warned — as part of their informed consent — that *retrograde ejaculation* is likely to occur afterwards, as a result of the removal in the course of the operation of the internal sphincter whose contraction normally prevents reflux of semen during ejaculation (see p. 236). In other respects their capacity to make love is not usually affected. Some patients may wish to postpone surgery for this reason when they are particularly anxious to have more children.

In *transurethral resection* of the prostate, a *resectoscope* is passed (Fig. 17.9), through which the operator first identifies the verumontanum and sphincter — the *landmarks* of the operation (Fig. 17.10). Then the

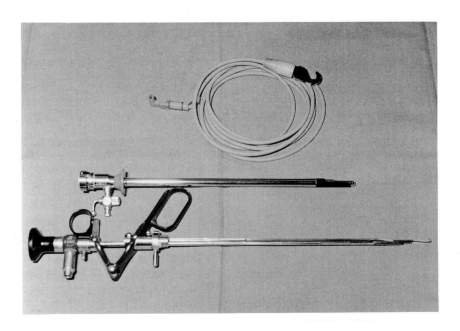

Fig. 17.9 A resectoscope: the loop cuts out the prostatic tissue with the arc of a cutting diathermy current, and seals bleeding vessels with the coagulating current.

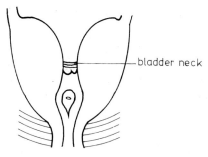

Fig. 17.10 In transurethral resection the operator starts by identifying the two 'landmarks' — the bladder neck fibres and the verumontanum.

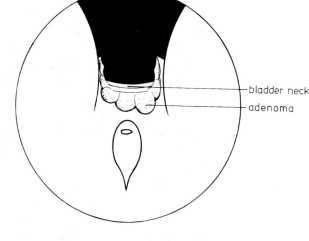

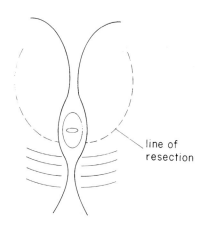

Fig. 17.11 If too much tissue is taken downstream of the verumontanum the supramembranous component of the sphincter mechanism may be destroyed, so care is taken always to preserve the verumontanum.

surgeon cuts away all the benign tissue, leaving behind the outer zone tissue — the 'capsule'. He takes care not to cut anything downstream of the verumontanum since below this landmark lies the all important supramembranous sphincter (Fig. 17.11).

After cutting out all the adenoma, the bleeding vessels are sealed off with the diathermy, and a three-way irrigating catheter is inserted (Fig. 17.12). This has to be larger than usual, (about 22 Ch) because it must accommodate an additional channel through which fluid is run in to dilute the blood that always continues to ooze from small vessels in the capsule.

Postoperative care after TUR prostate

The major hazard of prostatectomy is *haemorrhage* no matter how carefully the surgeon achieves haemostasis, so cross-matched blood must be available in case *transfusion* is required.

The *blood pressure* may have been lowered during the operation, and as it rises, reactionary haemorrhage is likely to occur from the small vessels in the prostatic capsule. The pulse and blood pressure are monitored every 15 to 30 minutes for the first few hours.

The *three-way Foley catheter* is left in the bladder with its balloon distended with 40 ml water. When there has been much bleeding, a Salvaris swab (Fig. 17.13) may have been tied round the catheter at its exit point to control venous bleeding by compression; it is usually left on for about 20 minutes to give time for blood to coagulate in the veins. If left on longer than an hour there is a risk of necrosis of the skin of the glans penis around the meatus.

The *three-way* catheter is irrigated continuously with normal saline at a rate which keeps the urine a pale pink colour. It is safer to use 1 litre bags, and empty the drainage after each litre has run through, rather than 3-litre containers. This also prevents the drainage bag from getting too full — for if it does, the non-return valve will be closed and the outflow from the bladder will be stopped (Fig. 17.14).

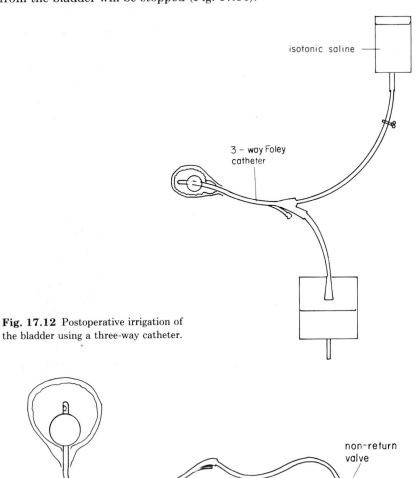

isotonic saline

3 – way Foley catheter

Fig. 17.12 Postoperative irrigation of the bladder using a three-way catheter.

non-return valve

increased pressure closes valve

Fig. 17.13 After transurethral resection a Salvaris swab may be used to compress the veins at the neck of the bladder; it must be removed after about 20 minutes to prevent a pressure sore from forming on the penis.

Fig. 17.14 If the drainage bag becomes overfull the non-return valve will be shut off; drainage bags should be emptied when they are about half full.

A very careful and accurate record must be kept of the volume of saline run in and out; obviously there should always be more coming out than goes in — since urine and blood will be added. If the total coming out is less than that run in then something has gone wrong. Check the following in order.

Blocked catheter.   Usually blockage is caused by a chip of prostate or a clot of blood. The patient will be in pain and his distended bladder can be felt suprapubically. If there is pain, this is the most likely cause, and the remedy is not to give an analgesic, but to unblock the catheter by:
1 Gently *'milking'* the catheter (Fig. 17.15).
2 If milking fails, the bladder should be *irrigated*. This calls for a strict aseptic technique (Fig. 17.16). Carefully clean the catheter connections with a spirit swab. Half fill a bladder syringe with saline, inject about 25 ml, and suck back firmly. A few clots will issue together with some urine, and the pressure in the bladder will be relieved. Continue to irrigate the

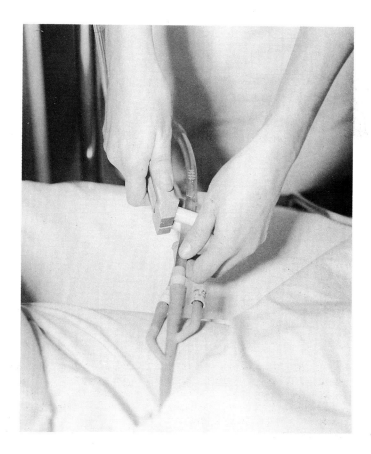

Fig. 17.15 Milking the catheter to remove obstructing blood clot.

bladder until no more clots are recovered, using only 25 ml at a time and always making sure that what is put in is sucked out. Reconnect the sterile bag.

3 If manual irrigation fails, the doctor will need to *change the catheter* and for this the patient will require an analgesic by injection. The catheter is often jammed with a fragment of prostate. If a free flow is obtained from the new catheter, the bladder is emptied and residual clot washed out with the bladder syringe.

4 If all these measures fail and the bladder remains distended with urine and clot the patient must be taken back to theatre at once. Under anaesthesia the resectoscope is again passed and the clot sucked out with the *Ellik evacuator* (Fig. 17.17), and the prostatic bed is searched for bleeding points which are coagulated with diathermy.

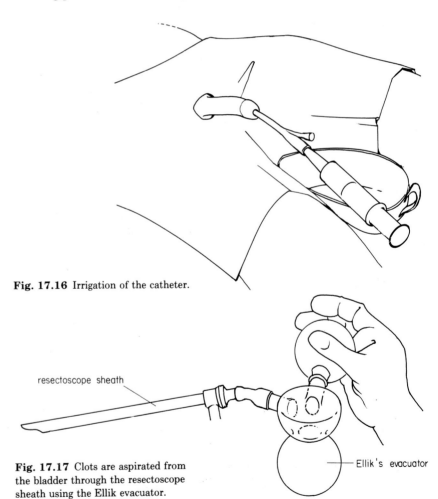

Fig. 17.16 Irrigation of the catheter.

resectoscope sheath

Ellik's evacuator

Fig. 17.17 Clots are aspirated from the bladder through the resectoscope sheath using the Ellik evacuator.

Extravasation of fluid into soft tissues or peritoneum. Fluid often escapes through the tiny holes that are made in the course of removing the adenoma from the capsule (Fig. 17.18) and the patient may have some tenderness in the pelvic area, different from the pain of clot retention which is due to the distension of the bladder. The medical staff must be informed. Small leaks are not serious; if the urine is only slightly bloodstained, the irrigation may be stopped — or its rate reduced. Catheter drainage will be continued for 4 or 5 days until the discomfort has settled.

Rarely there may be a large hole in the capsule with leakage of larger amounts of fluid causing more severe pain or even signs suggesting that the fluid has entered the peritoneal cavity. In such an event the patient is returned to theatre for the hole to be repaired through a suprapubic incision.

The TUR syndrome. Some fluid always enters the venous system through the holes made in the prostatic veins during the resection. It is only when a large volume escapes intravenously that danger arises. If water is used for the resection, the red cells may swell up and burst, releasing haemoglobin which chokes the renal tubules and leads to acute renal failure.

To prevent this danger, an isotonic fluid (such as glycine) is generally used for transurethral resection, but if an excess even of glycine enters the bloodstream the blood may be so diluted that the plasma sodium falls. This *hyponatraemia* results in disturbance of nerve conduction and muscle contraction. The patient may be very drowsy, experience transient blindness, have a fit, or appear to have had a stroke. Measurement of the

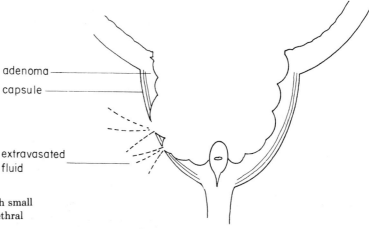

Fig. 17.18 Some irrigating fluid always leaks through small holes made in the outer zone 'capsule' during transurethral resection.

plasma sodium gives the diagnosis. A natural diuresis usually corrects the water overload within a few hours. Concentrated saline is sometimes given to restore the plasma sodium. The rate of irrigation is slowed to the minimum. Fits are controlled with anticonvulsants and frusemide may be given to help the patient get rid of the excess fluid.

Bacteraemia

Bacteraemia may strike without warning at any time in the first few days after TUR (see p. 48). It must be promptly recognized and treated as an emergency.

Hypotension

The blood pressure is often low immediately after the operation and unless he is breathless it is inadvisable to sit the patient up with more than two pillows until he has fully recovered from the anaesthetic and the bleeding has settled, or else the blood pressure may fall again dramatically.

Toilet of the catheter

A little discharge of blood and mucus around the catheter is inevitable and if neglected will form a stiff crust. It should be carefully wiped away to keep the patient comfortable and prevent infection. The day after the operation he can wash the area, using soap and water, himself and dry it carefully when necessary.

Paraphimosis

Check that the foreskin has been replaced or it may become trapped behind the glans penis, which then becomes swollen — paraphimosis — (Fig. 17.19). If this is noted the doctor should be informed at once for the sooner it is reduced the better.

Bladder spasm

As with other operations on the bladder, blood and urine may escape around the catheter from time to time; the patient will describe this as happening 'when I pass my water' (although he has a catheter in position). It is easy to jump to the conclusion that the catheter is blocked. Test it by clamping the catheter for a few seconds while the irrigation runs in and

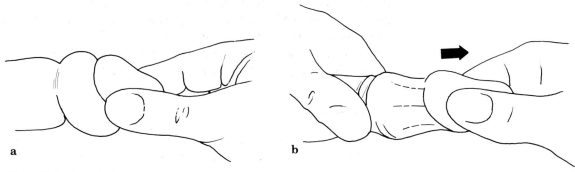

a   b

Fig. 17.19 If the foreskin is not
replaced after transurethral resection it
becomes painfully swollen —
'paraphimosis' should be reduced as soon
as possible.

then let it go; the irrigation will run out and one cannot palpate an
enlarged bladder. This is 'bladder spasm' (see p. 194) and is very common
after transurethral resection of the prostate. When he is up and about he
may seem to be behaving like a woman in labour — bending forward and
finding relief by deep breathing. He will require antispasmodics, analgesia
or diazepam, and most important of all — an explanation of what is
happening and assurance that nothing is wrong. Severe bladder spasms
may call for removal of the catheter somewhat earlier than would otherwise be desirable.

Early ambulation

The patient is encouraged to get up and walk around the ward on the day
after the operation, eat normally, and get used to drinking nearly 3 litres a
day which will dilute the urine and lessen the discomfort and the risk of
infection.

Antibiotic cover is given to men with pacemakers, artificial heart
valves and hip prostheses, and to those with known preoperative urinary
infection, and all those who have been catheterized for more than 24
hours. The appropriate antibiotic is given with the premedication, and
continued for 24 hours after the catheter has been removed.

Removal of the catheter

This is the big moment for the patient. The catheter is removed usually
about 2 days after the operation. It is always removed in the morning to
allow the patient to get used to controlling his urine again and to reduce
his intake towards the end of the day so that he gets some rest. Problems
are always easier to identify and solve in the day than at night.

The patient may be apprehensive, and an explanation of exactly what is going to happen and perhaps an analgesic beforehand will reduce this. He will feel more secure if he is provided with a urinal within reach, and a pad in case there is any dribbling or discharge of blood.

First make sure the catheter balloon is fully deflated by measuring the volume of water removed and checking that the tubing collapses when suction is applied to the balloon channel. (For the foley balloon that will not deflate, see p. 193.) Draw the catheter out gently and steadily into a receiver. There will be a moment of discomfort followed by a sense of relief. Some frequency and urgency must be expected at first as is the sensation of 'passing razor blades'. This usually settles quickly and good volumes are passed with a strong stream. A mid-stream urine is obtained; if infection is present it must be treated to minimize the risk of later secondary haemorrhage.

Before the patient goes home he is once more instructed to avoid exertion for the first two weeks, to drink 2 litres of fluid a day, and to expect to see a little blood reappearing in the urine about 10 days after the operation when the scab separates.

Failure to void

A few patients are unable to pass urine after the catheter has been removed, and if the bladder becomes distended the catheter must be replaced by the doctor. The patient will be disappointed but may be assured that a little more time may be needed to allow the swelling to go down. The catheter is usually taken out 2 or 3 days later, and the patient generally passes urine successfully the second time.

In a few cases the bladder fills up again. A catheter must be passed once more. It may be necessary to return the patient to theatre to make sure that all the obstructing tissue has been resected for it needs a surprisingly small amount of residual prostatic tissue to cause obstruction.

Sometimes the cause of the failure to void is not residual obstruction, but that the detrusor muscle has become so weakened by long over-distension that the bladder cannot empty itself. This is especially likely in men who have had long standing chronic retention. They tend to pass urine in small volumes, starting some hours after removal of the catheter, but the floppy bladder gradually fills up again. The bladder has to be allowed to rest for several weeks to recover its contractility.

A silicone rubber catheter is passed with a bag applied which can be worn unobtrusively under the clothing. These men can go home for 4 to 6 weeks, managing the catheter themselves with supervision from the community nurse if necessary. The patient and his carer must be shown, and practice, how to empty and change the bag, and will need a supply of spare bags to take home for changing weekly. Because they are often unable to concentrate their urine and will pass as much by night as by day, they need an extra bag which can be added on at night to accept this additional volume.

After 4 to 6 weeks at home, the patient is admitted for a day or two when the catheter is removed. A careful check is kept on urine output, and before he goes home the residual urine is measured with an ultrasound scan or a catheter to make sure the bladder is being emptied completely.

Incontinence

Occasionally the reverse is the outcome — the patient has no control over passing his urine. He becomes distressed or despondent, and tends to keep to his bed with a urinal in place. Such incontinence is rarely permanent and the patient should be encouraged. Carefully observe what is actually happening especially if he is incontinent when asleep — a less favourable sign. Encourage him to get up and look after himself — if necessary using incontinence pads and pants. Make sure that it is easy for him to get to the lavatory or a urinal and get him to try to pass urine at regular intervals. Exercising his perineal muscles by 'tucking in his tail' several times every hour may also help. Record and encourage his progress.

Sometimes the distal sphincter mechanism is rigid and cannot contract because it is infiltrated with prostatic carcinoma, and only when the tissues have become softer after a course of stilboestrol treatment (see below) does control return.

Very occasionally the sphincter mechanism is damaged by a technical error during the operation. These patients have total incontinence. The diagnosis is made by urodynamic studies and confirmed by urethroscopy which shows a defect in the ring of the sphincter muscle. None of the remedies for this distressing condition are really satisfactory (see p. 142). In the first instance the patient is provided with a condom or pubic pressure urinal to keep him comfortable and dry; later on implanting an artificial sphincter may be considered (see p. 139).

OPEN PROSTATECTOMY

There are several methods of open operation in use. The one favoured by most British urologists is *Millin's retropubic operation*. Through a Pfannenstiel incision (Fig. 17.20) the peritoneum is pushed back upwards away from the bladder and prostate and a transverse incision is made through the front of the capsule onto the adenoma (Fig. 17.21) which is

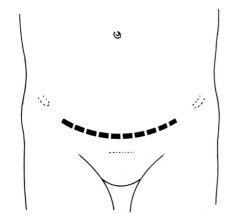

Fig. 17.20 The Pfannenstiel incision used for Millin's retropubic (open) prostatectomy.

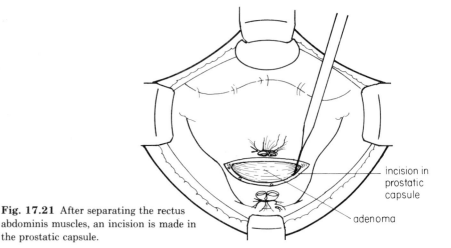

Fig. 17.21 After separating the rectus abdominis muscles, an incision is made in the prostatic capsule.

incision in prostatic capsule

adenoma

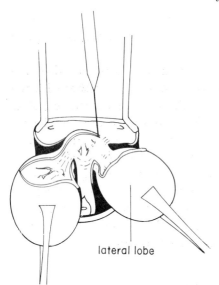

lateral lobe

Fig. 17.22 The inner zone 'adenoma' is shelled out.

shelled out of the capsule, leaving a cavity behind (Fig. 17.22). Bleeding is controlled by stitches and a catheter is inserted. Some surgeons use continuous irrigation, others prefer to leave the urine, mixed with blood, to drain away on its own.

In addition to the complications mentioned above for transurethral resection, open prostatectomy carries greater risks of wound and chest infection, deep vein thrombosis and pulmonary embolism; hazards which make any form of open prostatectomy more dangerous than transurethral resection. However, it has the advantage of requiring no specialized training or instruments, and of permitting the very largest glands to be removed. Even today in modern urological departments the open method is still used, though very rarely, when the prostate is too huge to be removed transurethrally.

Cancer of the prostate

In the outer zone of the prostate small foci of carcinoma are very common and will always develop if a man lives long enough. Indeed they are present in every male over the age of 80. It is only a small proportion of these which cause trouble by spreading outside the prostate.

When an early cancer of the prostate is discovered, as it may be by feeling a nodule in the prostate per rectum (Fig. 17.23) or detected by the laboratory in the tissue removed by transurethral resection for what was thought to be a benign gland, there is today a controversy as to the best form of treatment. There are three alternatives:

1 *Radical prostatectomy.* Many surgeons, especially in North America, feel that the entire gland should be removed by radical prostatectomy, an

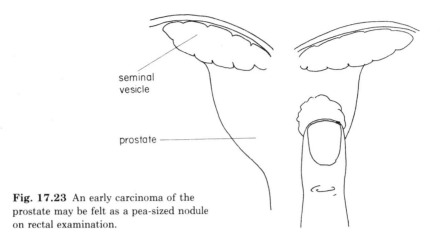

Fig. 17.23 An early carcinoma of the prostate may be felt as a pea-sized nodule on rectal examination.

operation which in skilled hands can be shown to give a life expectancy to the patient that is normal for his age, at the expense of the risk of some loss of continence and of potency.

2 *Radiotherapy.* In many centres, particularly in Britain, when the carcinoma is diagnosed it is treated with radiotherapy either with the linear accelerator or the implantation of radioactive gold or iodine grains.

3 *Deferred treatment.* Many surgeons have however noted that the life expectancy for men with this kind of small and incidentally found carcinoma of the prostate is so good that it is difficult to be sure that treatment either by surgery or radiotherapy is really going to improve matters. Instead they prefer to watch their patients carefully, and reserve treatment either for the carcinoma which comes back and causes urinary obstruction again, or begins to spread. It is probably true to say that this expectant treatment is the usual policy in Britain today.

Presentation of cancer of the prostate

In addition to these incidentally found cases, some men with urinary symptoms are found to have glands that are obviously hard and irregular on rectal examination. Their prostatic symptoms are corrected by a transurethral resection just as for the benign glands, but every effort is made to avoid performing any kind of open operation for fear of spreading the tumour into the wound.

Metastases from prostatic cancer

The common site for metastases from a primary carcinoma in the prostate are the bones where they cause backache and difficulty in walking. They are detected as 'hot spots' in a bone scan (Fig. 17.24) or as osteosclerotic deposits in an X-ray (Fig. 17.25). Cancer in the prostate may also spread to the liver and peritoneal cavity to cause ascites.

Acid phosphatase

The normal prostatic glands secrete this enzyme. Most prostatic cancers retain the ability to make this enzyme and when there is widespread cancer there is an excessive production of serum acid phosphatase and it spills over into the blood where it can be measured as the 'prostatic fraction' of the serum acid phosphatase.

Hormone control of the prostate

In lower mammals the prostate is one of those organs in the male — like the horns of the deer — which grow or shrink according to the mating season. This growth and shrinkage is caused by a rise and fall in the androgens produced in the testes. These changes can be started by giving androgens and stopped by removing the testicles or giving oestrogens.

About 80% of metastatic cancers of the prostate can be made to

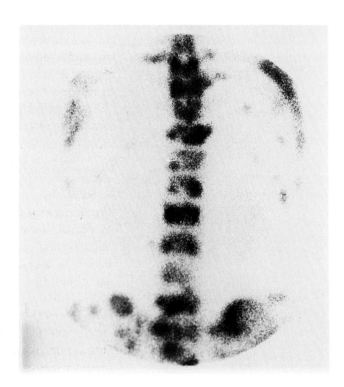

Fig. 17.24 An isotope bone scan showing areas of increased bloodflow caused by metastases of carcinoma of the prostate as 'hot spots'.

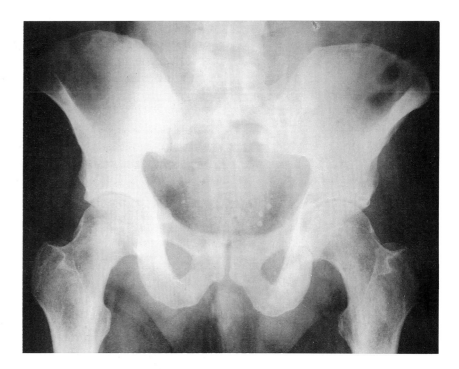

Fig. 17.25 An X-ray shows increased density in the bone where there are metastases of prostatic cancer.

resolve by removing the secretory part of the testicles — *subcapsular orchidectomy* with rapid and dramatic relief of pain. The same result may be achieved by giving oestrogens. These may be naturally occurring hormones such as ethinyl oestradiol, or the synthetic one stilboestrol (which is the cheapest and most effective). As all oestrogens have an increased risk of causing fluid retention and cardiovascular side-effects such as cardiac infarction or a stroke they are often contraindicated.

A tiny proportion of androgens are made in the adrenal, and sometimes when orchidectomy or stilboestrol has failed to control prostatic cancer one can obtain a response by giving drugs that stop the adrenal from making its own androgens, or drugs that block the action of androgens from any source on the prostatic cancer tissue.

Both the testes and the adrenals make their androgens at the orders of the pituitary. A new group of drugs — the luteinizing hormone-releasing hormone agonists (LHRH agonists) — overstimulate the pituitary until it is exhausted. For a few days testes and adrenals put out an excessive output of their androgens, and then stop. The effect is just as if both testicles and adrenal glands are removed. To start with there is a surge in the output of androgens and during this time metastases may enlarge and cause more pain which needs strong analgesics. Sometimes there are more serious side-effects, e.g. paraplegia from metastases in the spine. This is the dreaded 'LHRH flare'. It can be easily blocked by giving drugs which prevent androgen from affecting prostatic cancer cells. Such substances are cyproterone and flutamide. The combination of LHRH agonists and cyproterone or flutamide achieves a total androgen blockade without the cardiovascular side-effects of oestrogens and the slight discomfort of an orchidectomy.

In practice the results of this kind of medical androgen blockade are no better than simple subcapsular orchidectomy. The reason is that one in four cancers of the prostate are hormone resistant, and the three-quarters which start by being hormone sensitive, do not always remain so. They, and the original 25% are not controlled by androgens no matter whether they are formed in the testis or the adrenal. No variation on the theme of hormone therapy will cure them.

Radiotherapy

If metastases are localized, e.g. one or two painful metastases in a bone, radiotherapy will relieve pain and allow the bones to heal. This is especially useful when metastases in the vertebrae are compressing the spinal cord causing weakness of the legs and threatening paraplegia. A short course of radiotherapy may allow the patient to walk again if given promptly.

Chemotherapy

Chemotherapy has until recently been useless, and the newer combinations of platinum with other agents, though promising, must be regarded as still on trial.

Prostatitis

Acute prostatitis

There is a sudden onset of pain in the perineum with fever and sometimes rigors. The prostate gland is acutely swollen and tender to rectal palpation and the patient has pain and difficulty in passing urine. Microorganisms may be present together with pus in the urine. The inflammation usually resolves with prompt antibiotic treatment, analgesia and rest in bed, but if treatment is postponed an *abscess* may form, which gives rise to so much swelling of the gland that the patient cannot urinate at all. The abscess is drained through a resectoscope (Fig. 17.26) giving immediate relief; late and neglected cases may drain into the rectum and take longer to heal.

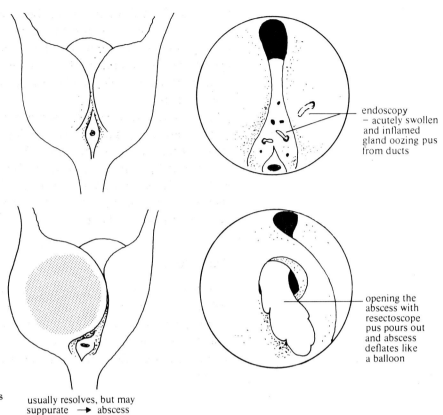

endoscopy – acutely swollen and inflamed gland oozing pus from ducts

opening the abscess with resectoscope pus pours out and abscess deflates like a balloon

usually resolves, but may suppurate ⟶ abscess

Fig. 17.26 Acute prostatitis usually resolves, but sometimes an abscess forms which is drained transurethrally.

Chronic prostatitis

Many patients have relapses of attacks of acute prostatitis which occur without warning, the first symptom being a rigor. In other patients there are vague symptoms of discomfort on voiding and in the perineum, and on rectal examination the prostate gland is found to be swollen and tender. If its secretions are expressed by *prostatic massage* one may find an excess of pus cells present, and the patient is labelled as suffering from chronic prostatitis. Seldom is there any real evidence of infection, and more often serious psychosomatic difficulties need to be evaluated.

Stones in the prostate

Small calculi are very common in the prostate between the two zones. They arise within dilated prostatic ducts, and although they may be accompanied by recurrent urinary infection, usually they are entirely innocent and do not need any treatment. Rarely a large group of stones in

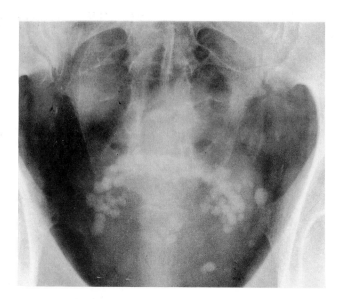

Fig. 17.27 Small stones are often found in the prostate.

the prostate (Fig. 17.27) may have to be removed. They are released with a resectoscope, pushed back into the bladder, and then removed by litholapaxy (see p. 85).

Further reading

Blandy, J. P. (1978) *Transurethral Resection*, 2nd edn. Pitman Medical, Tunbridge Wells.

Blandy, J. P. & Lytton, B. (eds) (1986) *The Prostate.* Butterworths, London.

Chisholm, G. D. (1985) Carcinoma of the prostate. In *Textbook of Genito-Urinary Surgery*, vol. 2, eds. Whitfield, H. N. & Hendry, W. F., pp. 1001–1018. Churchill Livingstone, Edinburgh.

Glode, L. M. (1985) Gonadotropin-releasing hormone analogues and other new hormonal treatments of prostate cancer. In *Genitourinary Cancer*, ed. Garnick, M. B., pp. 105–123. Churchill Livingstone, London.

Hinman, F. jr (ed.) (1983) *Benign Prostatic Hypertrophy*. Springer-Verlag, New York.

18 *The urethra*

The male urethra

Urethritis

Infective

GONORRHOEA

Gonorrhoea is the main cause of acute urethritis. The gram-negative intracellular diplococcus is acquired by sexual intercourse, and after a variable incubation period of 1 to 10 days there is a profuse urethral discharge of yellow-green pus and pain on passing water. Some patients may have very few symptoms and act as carriers. Neglected cases may be complicated by epididymitis (see p. 257) and prostatitis (see p. 218). It is important to make certain of the diagnosis by accurate identification of the organism by microscopy of the urethral discharge and culture of the *Neisseria gonorrhoeae.* Formerly universally sensitive to penicillin, many strains are today resistant to this antibiotic. Patients with gonorrhoea should be very carefully evaluated by those with special experience in sexually transmitted diseases in order not to miss infection with the more serious disease syphilis, and to make sure that contacts are diagnosed and treated before they develop serious complications. In the United Kingdom such patients should always be referred to a specialist department of genitourinary medicine.

NON-SPECIFIC URETHRITIS — NSU

Urethritis may be caused by a number of other infective agents such as the *Herpesvirus hominis, Trichomonas vaginalis,* and *Chlamydia trachomatis.* Clinically indistinguishable from gonorrhoea, the diagnosis requires careful laboratory tests. If the infection is caused by the parasite *Trichomonas vaginalis* it responds well to metronidazole. If the infection is caused by *Chlamydia,* there is usually a good response to treatment with the tetracyclines, but relapse is common, sometimes because of persistent infection in the prostate. In rare cases the serious complication — Reiter's disease — is seen, which gives rise to conjunctivitis, iritis and inflammation in the sacroiliac joints and spine.

221

Chemical urethritis

Sometimes the urethra will react to a catheter as if it were caustic and even after a relatively short period of catheterization there is a severe urethritis, pain on voiding, and a purulent discharge. Removing the catheter is very painful. It heals with a long stricture. Forty years ago this was caused by formaldehyde when it was used incorrectly to sterilize gum-elastic catheters. It was abolished when the formalin cabinet was banished from the hospital. Recent outbreaks of this condition in Australia and Finland have been traced to a toxic chemical used in the manufacture of latex rubber by one particular manufacturer. The condition tends to occur only in patients who have undergone cardio-vascular or aortic surgery.

Severe inflammation of the urethra from whatever cause will heal with a fibrous scar, and as elsewhere in the urinary tract, the scar will contract and give rise to a *stricture*. Post-gonococcal stricture was once common all over the world, but today is seen less often thanks to prompt and effective antibiotic treatment of acute urethritis.

Trauma to the urethra

Iatrogenic injury

The urethra has a very thin and delicate lining of epithelium which is easily torn by a stiff catheter or a cystoscope (Fig. 18.1). Sometimes these injuries are followed by a stricture.

Perineal injury

If a man falls astride a bar the urethra is forced up against the rigid inferior margin of the symphysis pubis (Fig. 18.2). The urethra may be partly or completely torn across, but the ends remain near each other because they are attached to the corpora cavernosa (Fig. 18.3). The danger is that urine will escape into the tissues of the perineum and cause sloughing of the overlying skin (Fig. 18.4). A suprapubic cystostomy is performed as an emergency (see p. 187). Later on a short stricture may form in the bulbar urethra (Fig. 18.5).

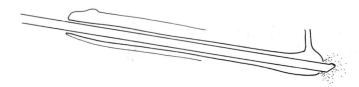

Fig. 18.1 The urethra is easily lacerated by a catheter or cystoscope.

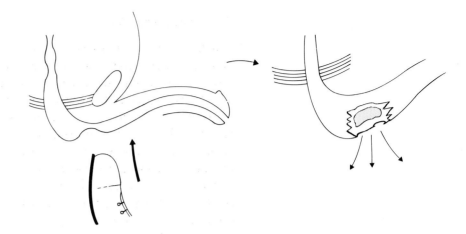

Fig. 18.2 A fall-astride or perineal injury lacerates the bulbar urethra.

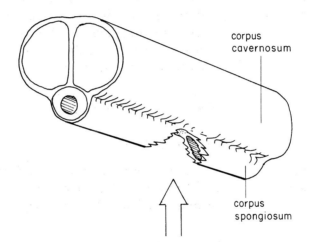

corpus cavernosum

corpus spongiosum

Fig. 18.3 In a perineal injury the ends of the urethra do not separate because they are splinted by the corpora cavernosa.

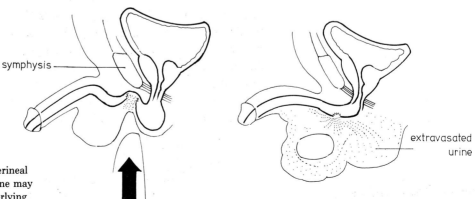

symphysis

extravasated urine

Fig. 18.4 The chief danger in perineal injury is that extravasation of urine may be followed by necrosis of the overlying skin and soft tissues.

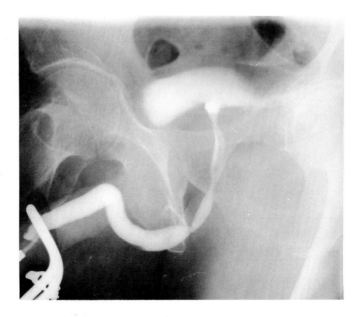

Fig. 18.5 A typical short bulbar stricture following perineal injury.

Fractured pelvis: ruptured membranous urethra

In some industrial and sports injuries the ring of the pelvis is compressed anteroposteriorly (Fig. 18.6) with the result that the thin rami of the pubis and ischium on either side of the symphysis are broken, and an X-shaped segment is carried backwards along with the bladder and prostate, tearing the urethra across at its weakest part — the membranous urethra. If the bony segment springs back to its former position, the ends of the urethra, if it has been torn right through, are near each other and if there is a stricture, it is a short one (Fig. 18.7).

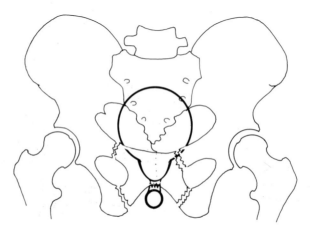

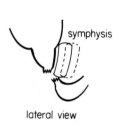

symphysis

lateral view

Fig. 18.6 The common type of fractured pelvis where the symphysis is forced backwards displacing the prostatic urethra.

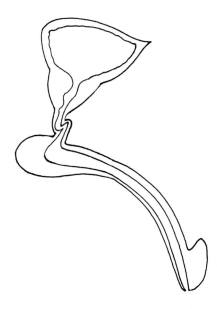

Fig. 18.7 The typical short S-shaped stricture that follows the usual type of fractured pelvis.

In other, more serious types of pelvic fracture, one-half of the pelvis is displaced upwards with a fracture dislocation of the sacro-iliac joint as well as another in the front of the pelvic ring (Fig. 18.8). Sometimes it is impossible to effect a perfect reduction of this fracture, so that the severed ends of the urethra are held apart. These patients are often young and seriously ill from other and more important injuries of the head, liver, spleen or chest. A suprapubic cystostomy is performed (see p. 187) as an emergency measure but as soon as they are sufficiently well the ends of the urethra must be brought together by an open operation, or there will be a very long and difficult stricture needing *urethroplasty* (see p. 229).

Urethral stricture

Congenital

POSTERIOR URETHRAL VALVES

These are common in new born children. A thin membrane shaped like a parachute obstructs the urine just below the verumontanum and causes gross obstruction to the bladder, ureters and kidneys (Fig. 18.9). The diagnosis may be made at birth or in early childhood, depending on the completeness of the obstruction. The child may strain so much to pass urine that he defaecates — 'he dirties when he wees'. Some babies are

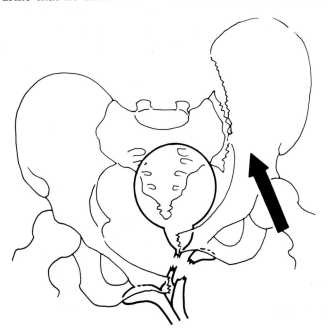

Fig. 18.8 In the more serious fracture of the pelvis one entire half of the pelvis is forced upwards, carrying the prostate and bladder with it. The severed ends of the urethra are held apart by the displaced bony fragments.

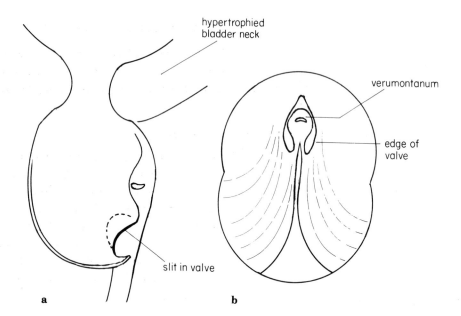

Fig. 18.9 Congenital posterior urethral valves.

born with grossly obstructed ureters and kidneys. The diagnosis is made with a cystogram, and the valves are divided with a paediatric resectoscope. The gross dilatation of the upper tracts which has occurred *in utero* may never recover completely.

ANTERIOR URETHRAL VALVES

These are rare. A second urethra lies under the normal one, separated by a thin membrane with a perforation in it. When the little boy passes water, the second urethra balloons out and the membrane acts like a valve to prevent urine getting out (Fig. 18.10). The valve-like membrane is divided by a tiny knife passed through the paediatric resectoscope. Occasionally the urethra must be reconstructed if it remains too big and baggy.

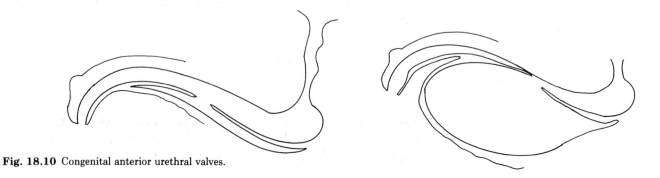

Fig. 18.10 Congenital anterior urethral valves.

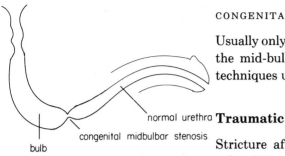

normal urethra

congenital midbulbar stenosis

bulb

Fig. 18.11 Congenital midbulbar stenosis.

Usually only noticed when the young man grows up, there is a tight ring in the mid-bulbar urethra (Fig. 18.11). It is easily treated by any of the techniques used in treating urethral strictures.

Traumatic

Stricture after perineal injury is always short. After fractures of the pelvis it involves the membranous urethra and is easy to treat if there has been only a slight displacement of the ends of the urethra, but very difficult to put right if the ends are far apart and no effort has been made to get them together. In either type, the fracture of the pelvis also tears across the small nerves and arteries that are necessary for normal erection and about half of these patients are made impotent by the injury. Naturally this is very distressing and patients need counselling.

Inflammatory strictures

These usually involve long lengths of the urethra, in gonorrhoea it is the bulb which is usually involved because here the paraurethral glands are most numerous. They may present many years after the long forgotten episode of urethritis, with a poor stream, acute retention or recurrent urinary infections.

Investigation

Strictures are investigated by means of a *urethrogram* (Fig. 18.12). Contrast medium is injected into the urethra to define the narrow part. The contrast medium is very hypertonic and the investigation is uncomfortable, so analgesics should be given beforehand. For the same reason the urethra remains very sore afterwards and it is painful to pass urine for a few hours.

Treatment of a urethral stricture

DILATATION

The stricture is stretched by passing flexible or rigid steel dilators (Fig. 18.13) which come in sets of gradually increasing size, marked in Charrière sizes. These dilators are sometimes called *sounds* because they

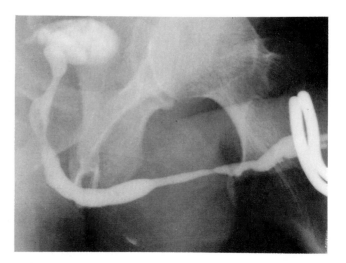

Fig. 18.12 Urethrogram showing anterior stricture.

used to be used to diagnose stones in the bladder by 'sounding' for them and sometimes *bougies* because they used to be made like candles, out of wax, and the best wax was imported to France from Bougia, near Algiers. When the stricture is very narrow, a thin *filiform* bougie (French, fil=thread) is passed first, and dilators of increasing size are screwed on to the end of the filiform (Fig. 18.14). Dilatation is usually performed in the outpatient department under local anaesthetic.

After explaining what is going to happen, the patient lies flat. The penis is cleaned with cetrimide and the urethra is filled with 1% lignocaine anaesthetic gel, which is kept in place with a penile clamp (see Figs. 16.12 and 16.13) for 5 minutes. The bougies are then gently passed, each one larger than the next, until the surgeon judges that the stricture has been stretched enough, his object being to stretch the scar tissue, not to tear it.

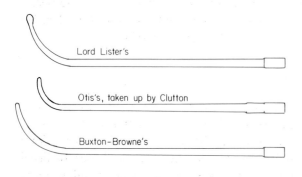

Lord Lister's

Otis's, taken up by Clutton

Buxton-Browne's

Fig. 18.13 Dilators or urethral 'sounds'.

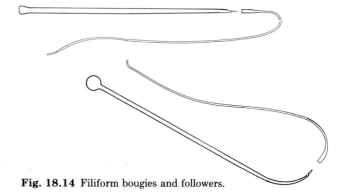

Fig. 18.14 Filiform bougies and followers.

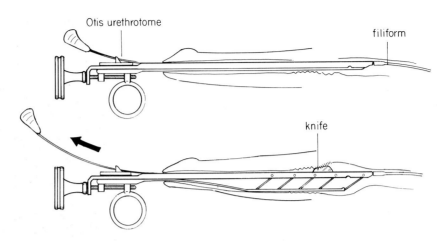

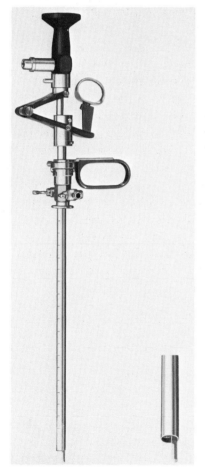

Fig. 18.15 The Otis urethrotome.

Fig. 18.16 Sachse optical urethrotome.

INTERNAL URETHROTOMY

The stricture is slit open from within with the *Otis urethrotome* (Fig. 18.15) or the *Sachse optical urethrotome* (Fig. 18.16). A silicone catheter is left in for a few days after urethrotomy to prevent extravasation of urine. Urethrotomy is usually performed under general anaesthesia, and the patient is warned that a catheter will be left in afterwards.

URETHROPLASTY

Preoperative preparation

When the operation is explained to the patient he will understand the need for a *thorough shave* of the pubic and perineal areas and will understand that he will be more comfortable if he has had a good *bowel action.* He must anticipate wearing a urethral *catheter* for 2 weeks and there may also be a suprapubic one while healing takes place. The genital area will be sore and bruised for a few days, and the dressings are rather bulky so that activity is reduced. Analgesics will be given if needed. He should expect to be away from work for about 6 weeks.

ISLAND PATCH URETHROPLASTY

Many operations have been devised for the permanent cure of a bad urethral stricture. One reliable technique makes a patch from the loose skin of the scrotum which is provided with a vascular pedicle made from the dartos muscle which lies under the skin. These dartos pedicled patches can be used to provide a permanent enlargement for almost any stricture in the urethra (Fig. 18.17).

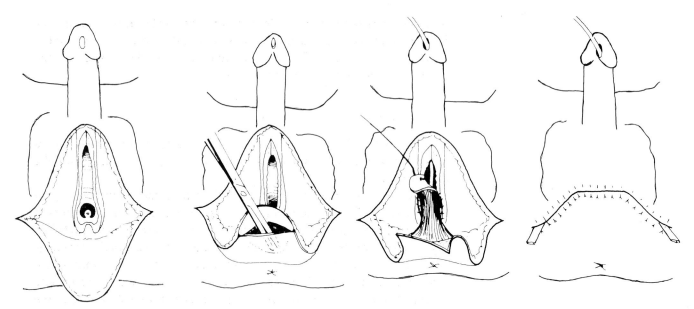

Fig. 18.17 A patch of scrotal skin on a vascular pedicle of dartos muscle is used to enlarge the urethra.

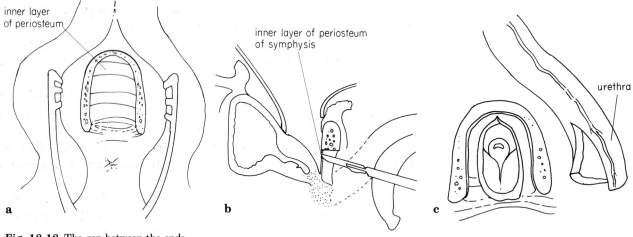

Fig. 18.18 The gap between the ends of the urethra after a displaced fracture of the pelvis is bridged by making (a) a window in the symphysis pubis, through which (b and c) the mobilized bulbar urethra is brought.

END TO END ANASTOMOSIS

For the strictures that follow rupture of the membranous urethra, when there is no displacement, the bulbar urethra is mobilized and anastomosed to the lower end of the prostatic urethra, having cut through the scar tissue.

When there is a wide gap between the prostatic and the bulbar urethra, because it has not been possible to reduce the displacement of the bony fracture, it is necessary to cut a window out of the inferior margin of the symphysis, before the bulbar urethra can be joined to the lower end of the urethra without any tension (Fig. 18.18).

Postoperative care

After the operation the penis is encased in a light compressive foam dressing which remains in place for 2 to 3 days to prevent formation of a haematoma.

There will be a perineal wound, usually with a soft drain discharging into a dressing. Considerable oozing during the first 24 to 48 hours make it necessary to change the outer dressings before they become soaked. When the drains are taken out 48 hours or so after operation the bulky dressings are removed, the area is examined for haematoma and bruising, and a smaller dressing applied. By the following day the leakage has usually reduced to a little serous fluid and the patient can take a shower or saline bath. An effective means of keeping the perineal area as dry as possible is a hand held hair-drier. A clean dry dressing is kept in place with elastonet pants. The sutures are usually removed after 10 days. The patient will appreciate a soft cushion or an air ring to sit on when he gets up, but lying or standing are usually more comfortable positions.

Because of the risk of anaerobic infection in a wound so close to the anus, prophylactic antibiotics are given in the early postoperative period, at first intravenously.

The urethral and (if one is used) suprapubic catheters are both allowed to drain freely all the time and either or both may do so. Care must be taken to prevent them being pulled on by securing them carefully. A fluid balance chart is recorded and the patient is encouraged to drink 3 litres of fluid to reduce the risk of infection. Daily catheter specimens of urine are taken for culture.

The urethral catheter is usually removed after 14 days. It is removed very slowly and gently, being careful to ensure that the balloon is completely deflated so as not to damage the skin graft area in the urethra. If present, a suprapubic catheter is clamped off at the same time.

There is unlikely to be any difficulty in voiding, but the suprapubic tube is released if necessary. If all is well the suprapubic tube is removed next day and a firm dressing applied. The site heals very rapidly.

Occasionally there is a leak of urine through a small hole in the perineal wound. The patient should be forewarned of this possibility or otherwise he may be distressed and fear that 'it has all gone wrong'. Assure him that there is no cause for alarm; these tiny fistulae heal of their own accord. Light finger pressure on the little hole when urine is being passed will keep him dry and the little fistula will dry up within a few days.

When it is healed, the skin graft does not empty out like the normal urethra does, and the patient should be taught how to express the teaspoonful or so of urine that remains there each time he urinates by milking forward. This will prevent dribbling.

Late complications

As time goes by the skin graft may grow and form an even larger pocket which must be trimmed. Hairs continue to grow, and if there is any obstruction, 'hairball stones' may form on them and require endoscopic removal.

Impotence

A young man with a stricture following a fractured pelvis is often (and rightly) concerned about the possibility of *impotence* having noted that he has had no erections since his injury. It may take up to 2 years before the normal mechanism of erection recovers, but at first it is important to give him the opportunity to express his worries and discuss them with the surgeon. Fortunately modern treatments are very effective if spontaneous recovery does not take place (see p. 237).

Cancer of the urethra

Primary cancer may occur in the urethra upstream of a chronic stricture. It is rare and has usually spread into the inguinal lymph nodes by the time it is first discovered. It is removed by total excision of the urethra, usually after a preliminary course of radiotherapy.

Secondary cancer occurs from primary lesions in the bladder that have seeded themselves in the urethra. It is one reason why cystourethrectomy should be performed. Sometimes superficial lesions can be controlled with the Neodymium YAG laser.

The female urethra

Diseases of the female urethra

Urethritis

Acute urethritis is often part of the common lower urinary tract infection of otherwise healthy women. It gives severe pain on voiding. The cause is usually *Escherichia coli* and it usually responds promptly to antibiotics.

Chronic urethritis also occurs, sometimes with dilatation and the accumulation of infected debris in the paraurethral glands. In addition to appropriate antibiotics, dilatation of the urethra under anaesthesia may help to empty the glands and shorten the course of the disease.

A paraurethral abscess may form when a gland is obstructed and infected. It is like a boil on the skin, and can be equally painful. Pus may be squeezed out if the urethra is stroked forwards. Rarely they need to be drained under anaesthesia.

Urethral diverticula

Larger pockets are sometimes found in the urethra; some are undoubtedly of congenital origin, lying either side of the midline (Fig. 18.19) and stones may form in them. They are excised through a 'trapdoor' incision in the vaginal wall (Fig. 18.20). A pack is placed in the vagina after the operation which is gently removed after 48 hours. A catheter remains *in situ* for 10 to 14 days to allow the urethra to heal.

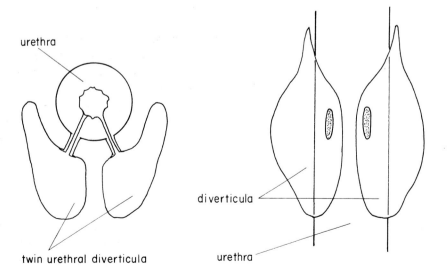

Fig. 18.19 Female urethral diverticula may be single or double.

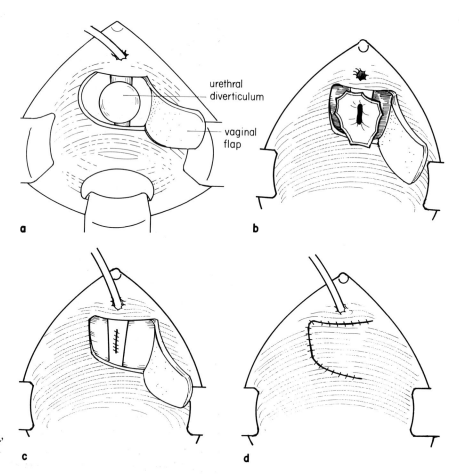

urethral
diverticulum

vaginal
flap

a

b

c

d

Fig. 18.20 Removal of a female
urethral diverticulum through a 'trapdoor'
incision in the vagina.

Caruncle

This confusing term covers four quite different conditions and should
really never be used.

1 Prolapse of the urethral mucosa (Fig. 18.21). A rim of pink tissue is
seen at the urethral orifice. It needs no treatment.

2 A thrombosed vein under the mucosa of the urethra may protrude out
of the urethral orifice like a thrombosed pile from the anal canal
(Fig. 18.22). If seen early on it can be very painful but is easily removed
under anaesthesia. When seen late it is better left to resolve on its own.

3 A benign angioneuroma may occur in the mucosa of the urethral
orifice: bright red, very painful and bleeding when touched. It should be
excised to make sure that it is not a carcinoma.

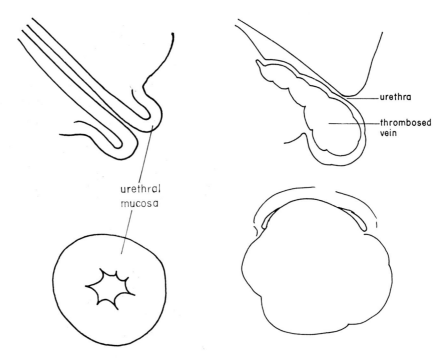

Fig. 18.21 Prolapsed urethral mucosa.   **Fig. 18.22** Thrombosed urethral vein.

4 Urethral carcinomas in women arise in the paraurethral glands and recur locally unless widely excised. To perform an excision that will get really clear of the tumour, it may be necessary to remove the bladder neck and sphincter mechanism and in such a case there is no point in trying to keep the bladder. Cystectomy may be performed with urinary diversion by means of an ileal conduit (see p. 173). Radiotherapy is given after the surgical removal but unfortunately the prognosis is very poor.

Further reading

Blandy, J. P. (1986) *Operative Urology*, 2nd edn, pp. 206–233. Blackwell Scientific Publications, Oxford.

Blandy, J. P. (1980) Urethral stricture. *Postgraduate Medical Journal*, **56**, 383–418.

Bracken, R. B. (1982) Exenterative surgery for posterior urethral cancer. *Urology*, **19**, 248–251.

Woodhouse, C. R. J., Flynn, J. T., Molland, E. A. & Blandy, J. P. (1980) Urethral diverticula in females. *British Journal of Urology*, **52**, 305–310.

19 *The penis*

Anatomy

The penis is made of three spongy units, the two corpora cavernosa and the corpus spongiosum which encloses the male urethra and ends in the glans penis (Fig. 19.1). The three erectile bodies are enclosed in a tough sleeve — Buck's fascia.

Erection and ejaculation

In erection blood is shunted into the corpora, tightly filling them with blood until they become rigid.

At the moment of ejaculation the bladder neck contracts under the control of the sympathetic nerves to the bladder, preventing semen from refluxing into the bladder. There are two phases in ejaculation:
1 the vas deferens and its ampulla contract and empty about 0.5 ml of live sperms into the prostatic urethra;
2 the seminal vesicles squirt about 4 ml of additional fluid to flush the sperms out of the erect urethra (Fig. 19.2).

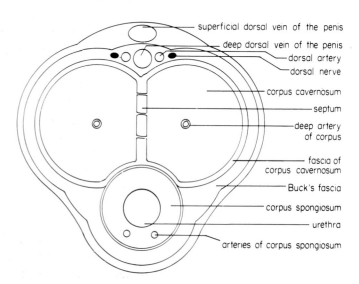

Fig. 19.1 Cross-section through the penis.

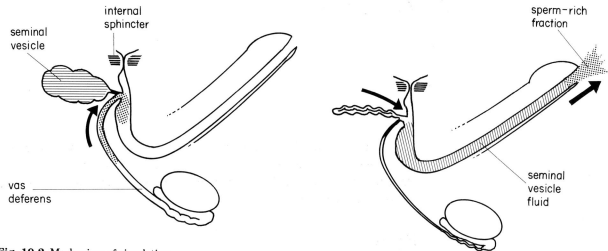

Fig. 19.2 Mechanism of ejaculation.

Impotence

Erectile impotence

In erectile impotence there is a failure of the cavernous tissue of the three erectile bodies to fill with blood either because the blood supply is blocked, or the nervous control of the blood supply is damaged.

The arteries of the penis (Fig. 19.1) spring from the internal pudendal branch of the internal iliac artery and they can be obstructed at any level by atheroma — the inevitable sequel of old age — by the arterial changes of diabetes, by surgical operations which involve ligature of the internal iliac arteries and by fractures of the pelvis. Impairment of the arterial blood supply may be shown by Doppler studies of the penile blood flow, and the level of the obstruction can be exactly pinpointed by pelvic angiography.

The blood flow into the penis is under the control of the autonomic nervous system. The parasympathetic nerves may be diseased in diabetes, or injured in a fracture of the pelvis or during the removal of a cancer of the bowel. When they are damaged the normal shunting of blood into the penis cannot take place even though the arteries are patent.

Brindley's test

Recently a more simple test has been introduced to show whether or not the blood supply is impaired. A painless drug — papaverine — which causes the penile arteries to relax is injected directly into the penis and produces an erection so long as the blood supply is not obstructed. When successful, this not only becomes a diagnostic test — but also a way of treatment. The patient or his wife can inject the penis in the privacy of their home and restore the ability to make love.

Ejaculatory impotence

Ejaculatory impotence may be caused by damage to the sympathetic nerves in the pelvis or the internal sphincter at the neck of the bladder.

Sympathetic nerve damage

When the sympathetic ganglia or their nerves are injured in the course of operations on the aorta, or node dissection for testicular cancer, the seminal vesicles are paralysed and the bladder neck does not contract to prevent reflux of semen into the bladder. Some alpha-blocking drugs given for hypertension have a similar effect.

Damage to the bladder neck

Some men are born with a defect in the neck of the bladder which prevents it from contracting, and others have undergone surgical incision of the neck of the bladder to overcome retention of urine. After prostatectomy, for example, reflux of semen almost always takes place. In such patients semen can be recovered from the urine and used for artificial insemination.

Psychogenic impotence

In many instances there is nothing wrong with the anatomy of the penis or its blood supply, but there is a psychological problem for which expert psychosexual counselling may provide a remedy. When there is doubt one may perform 'nocturnal tumescence studies'. Erections occur several times during the night during the specially deep sleep which is accompanied by rapid eye movements. A pair of simple strain gauges are attached to the penis to record increases both in the circumference and the length of the penis. The recorder runs all through the night (Fig. 19.3). Paper strips put on by the patient in the privacy of his bedroom give much the same information at far less cost (Fig. 19.4).

Treatment

When the blood supply is intact, the patient may inject himself with

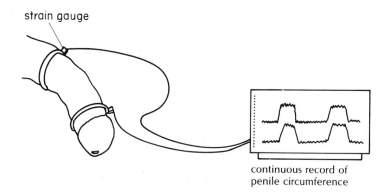

strain gauge

continuous record of
penile circumference

Fig. 19.3 Apparatus for recording
nocturnal penile tumescence.

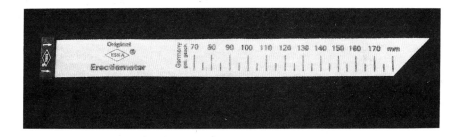

Fig. 19.4 Paper strips used to measure
and record nocturnal penile tumescence.

papaverine as described above. When the blood supply is blocked it is
occasionally possible to bypass the blockage and restore a normal blood
supply.

When there are perfectly good nocturnal erections the patient may be
cured by psychotherapy in the hands of a psychiatrist interested in the
condition.

For the remaining patients all hope is not lost. It is possible to provide
an artificial method of obtaining an erection by means of a penile
prosthesis.

Penile prostheses

Semi-stiff rods of silicone rubber may be placed inside the corpora
cavernosa to make them permanently semi-erect (Fig. 19.5). A modifi-
cation of this has a silver wire inside which can be bent and unbent many
times to allow the patient to tuck his penis away (Fig. 19.6). Scott's latest
device is much more sophisticated (Fig. 19.7) the cylinders in the corpora
can be pumped up or let down by manipulation of a little valve placed in
the scrotum.

All these devices have the inevitable defects of any implanted foreign
body; they tend to be extruded, to attract infection and to break in use, but

when successful can be of great value especially to the young diabetic and the young victim of a pelvic fracture. Their main disadvantage is that they are inordinately expensive.

The most important factor governing success or failure is infection. Every possible precaution must be taken to prevent infection — the skin must be carefully shaved and prepared before operation. Prophylactic

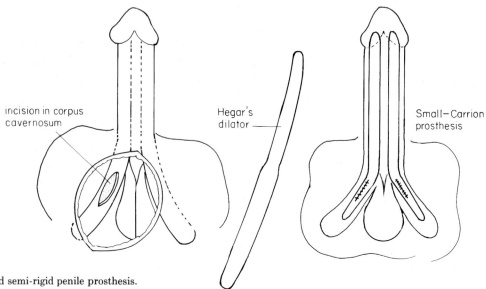

incision in corpus cavernosum

Hegar's dilator

Small–Carrion prosthesis

Fig. 19.5 Insertion of standard semi-rigid penile prosthesis.

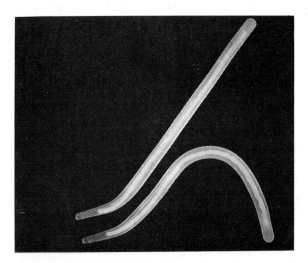

Fig. 19.6 Jonas' flexible penile prosthesis.

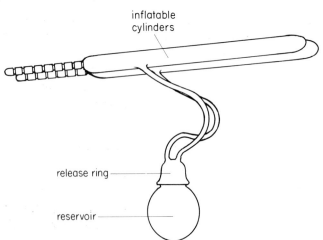

inflatable cylinders

release ring

reservoir

Fig. 19.7 Inflatable penile prosthesis (Surgitek Uniflate 1000 ®).

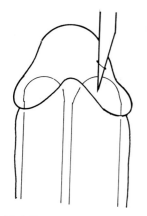

Fig. 19.8 Priapism: incision to allow blood to flow from the corpora cavernosa into the corpus spongiosum.

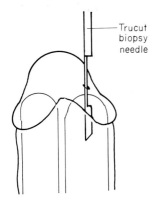

— Trucut biopsy needle

Fig. 19.9 Using a Trucut biopsy needle to make a window between the corpora cavernosum and spongiosum.

antibiotics are used in every case, and the prosthesis itself is soaked in an antibiotic solution before being implanted into a wound that has been irrigated with antibiotics. The patient is warned to postpone 'activation' of the appliance until the tissues around it have had time to heal completely.

Priapism

This is a surgical emergency in which an erection will not subside and is distressing for the patient. It is seen in blood disorders such as sickle cell disease and leukaemia and in patients undergoing dialysis, but the majority have no obvious cause. The blood does not coagulate in the corpora cavernosa, but it becomes very thick — like jam.

When seen early it can be reversed by injection of adrenaline or aramine. If this fails, it may be necessary to bypass the blocked channels by making a hole between the flaccid corpus spongiosum and one or other of the corpora cavernosa using a knife (Fig. 19.8), a biopsy needle (Fig. 19.9) or by making a surgical anastomosis between them (Fig. 19.10). If these simple measures fail one may decompress the corpora cavernosa by anastomosing one of them to the saphenous vein (Fig. 19.11).

Hypospadias

This is a common congenital anomaly affecting the penis to a varying extent (Fig. 19.12). In the most common form — glandular hypospadias, there is really no need to do anything, though if parents insist, the meatus advancement glanuloplasty (MAGPI) operation (Fig. 19.13) gives a normal-looking penis and can be done as a day case.

In more severe deformities there is shortening of the urethra and curvature of the penis (chordee) and it is necessary to straighten the urethra. Today this may be done in a single operation (Fig. 19.14). Operations for hypospadias are postponed until the child is out of nappies, but should be completed before he goes to infant school.

Nursing care

Parents can assist greatly in the preparation for surgery and aftercare and the child should be able to understand a simple explanation of what is going to happen, using words with which he is familiar.

The operation will only involve the penis and the surgeon will apply secure dressings to avoid any damage and to prevent the catheter from being dislodged. The child is kept on his bed as a further precaution, and

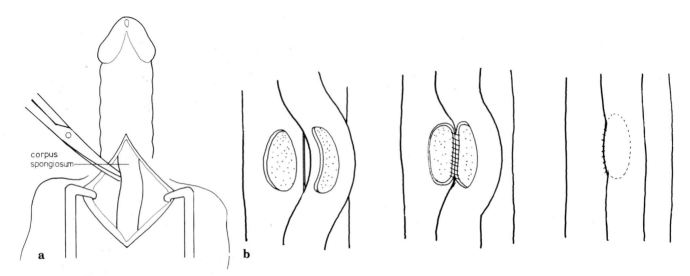

corpus
spongiosum

a   b

Fig. 19.10 Corpus–corpus shunt.

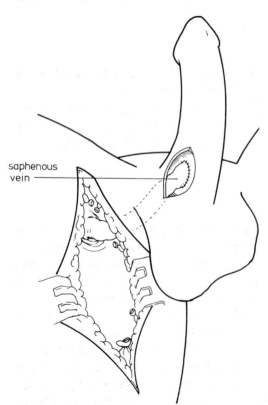

saphenous
vein

Fig. 19.11 Corpus–saphenous shunt.

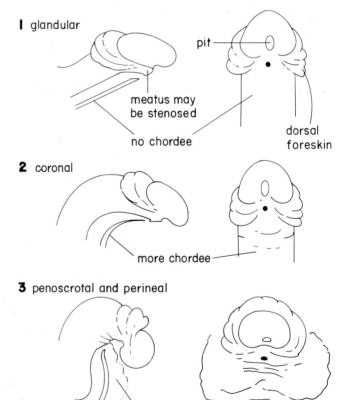

1 glandular

pit

meatus may
be stenosed

no chordee

dorsal
foreskin

2 coronal

more chordee

3 penoscrotal and perineal

short sharply curved penis with marked chordee

Fig. 19.12 Hypospadias occurs in a varying degree of severity.

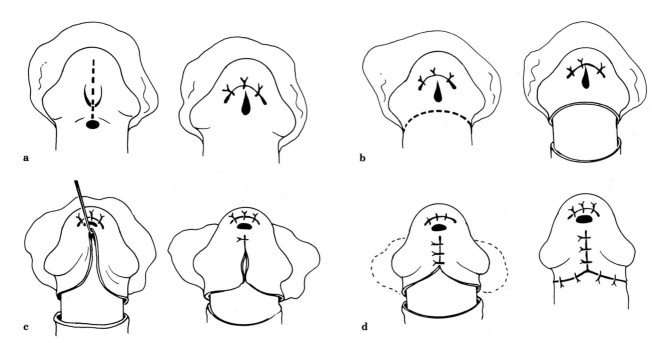

Fig. 19.13 Meatus advancement
glanduloplasty (MAGPI) operation.

needs to be occupied. Light arm restraint should only be used if really necessary to prevent him from pulling at his dressings.

The surgeon will give instructions about the removal of the catheter and sutures (unless absorbable ones are used). When and if they must be removed, a parent or a favourite nurse at hand can divert his attention or comfort him.

Circumcision

The foreskin probably serves quite a useful function in infancy, protecting the meatus from irritation by ammonia from urine soaked napkins. It is normal for the foreskin not to be fully separated from the glans penis until the age of 3 years, but after that, if the foreskin cannot be drawn back to keep the glans free of smegma, circumcision should be considered. Before that time it should not be meddled with and attempts to retract the foreskin before the age of 2 or 3 should be discouraged.

Later on, if the foreskin cannot be drawn back (*phimosis*) irritation develops under its hood, causing *balanitis*, and repeated episodes of balanitis probably act as a predisposing cause of cancer of the penis, rare though this disease is in the West. For this reason circumcision is advised whenever it is impossible to keep the glans clean by ordinary soap and water.

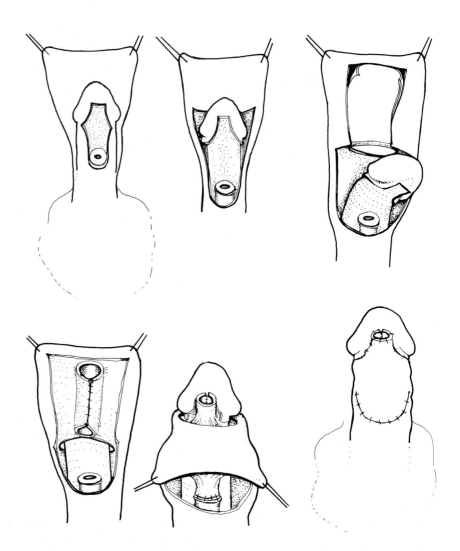

Fig. 19.14 One-stage operation for hypospadias.

The operation is performed under general anaesthesia. The foreskin is removed and after securing perfect haemostasis the inner and outer edges are sewn together with very fine catgut (Fig. 19.15).

The child will spend very little time in hospital. He must be carefully observed for bleeding, and one should make sure he has passed urine after the operation. If a dressing has been used it may be soaked off in a warm bath. Pants should be used which do not chafe and may easily be changed if soiled.

In adults circumcision is a more serious procedure, indicated when the foreskin cannot be retracted and especially when there is any suspicion of cancer — which is always suspect when the glans cannot be inspected.

In adults the prepuce may be so adherent to the glans that when it is

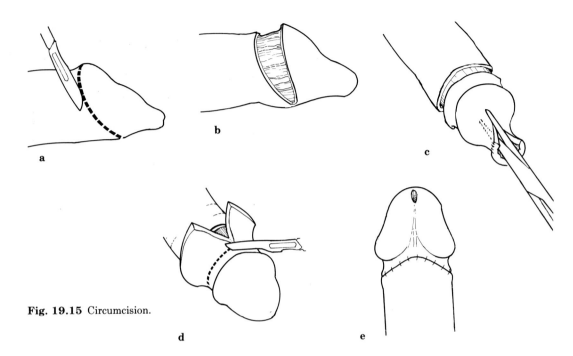

Fig. 19.15 Circumcision.

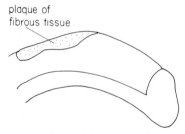

Fig. 19.16 Peyronie's disease: plaques of fibrous tissue form in the fascia of the penis.

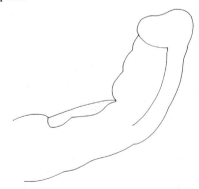

Fig. 19.17 In erection the plaque fails to expand and a bend forms in the penis.

dissected away the glans is left raw and bleeding; a vaseline gauze dressing is applied. It may take a week or so before the glans grows a new protective cover of skin, during which time comfortable loose cotton pants, frequent saline dressings and reduced activity are needed. The patient needs to be reassured that the penis will eventually come to look entirely normal.

Paraphimosis

When a catheter is put in for whatever reason, it is important to make sure that the foreskin is drawn back over the glans, otherwise it gets stuck (paraphimosis) behind the glans which swells and the surrounding tissues become so oedematous that the foreskin can only be replaced with a general anaesthetic. Before this stage is reached the paraphimosis may be reduced if the glans is pulled out to elongate it and make it narrower, so as to allow the foreskin to be replaced (see p. 211).

Peyronie's disease

Hard plaques of fibrous tissue form in the fascia of the penis (Fig. 19.16) and in erection prevent the penis from distending (Fig. 19.17). The condition is benign and it gets better if left alone though the improvement may take months or even years. Nobody knows its cause; nobody has a good treatment for it. If the penis is so bent that coitus is impossible, the bend may be corrected by taking a reef in Buck's fascia on the side opposite to the plaque — *Nesbit's operation* (Fig. 19.18).

Carcinoma of the penis

This is never seen in men circumcised in infancy, and is very rare in those who can easily retract and keep the glans penis clean.

It usually starts in the foreskin or glans penis, and later spreads down into the shaft of the penis, metastasizing to the lymph nodes of the groins. In its early stages (Fig. 19.19) it is treated by circumcision followed by local radiotherapy. If it is invading the shaft of the penis, or if the growth returns a few years later, amputation is needed.

Nursing care

Amputation of the penis causes deep-seated distress to a man who feels he is losing the symbol of his manhood, but where there is a loving marital relationship it is possible to work through these fears and come to terms with the situation, especially if the partners are aware of the alternative.

For someone on his own, the feeling of being less than a man may be

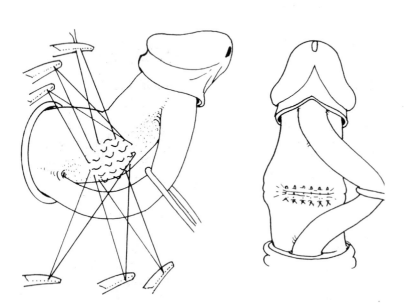

Fig. 19.18 Reefing operation to correct the bend in Peyronie's disease.

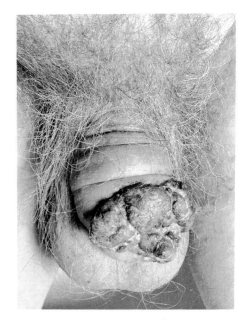

Fig. 19.19 Carcinoma of the penis confined to the glans; penis may be treated with radiotherapy.

more than he can tolerate. He must be able to express his feelings, and the help of a psychiatrist may be most valuable. Privacy is necessary when the operation is discussed or and when examinations and dressings are being performed. A nurse must be particularly careful not to communicate any emotional reaction at the sight of the wound, by action or facial expression. It is also very necessary to understand and respect the wishes of the patient as to whether he wants to see or feel the area.

Partial amputation

Fortunately most amputations of the penis remove only the distal few centimetres of the penis (Fig. 19.20) and when it is healed up men are able to obtain satisfactory erection, penetration and orgasm with what is left behind, and are usually able to pass urine in the standing position.

Total amputation

When the growth has spread to the proximal parts of the corpora cavernosa or has started to grow into the scrotum, it is usual to remove the contents of the scrotum along with the penis. The result is a perineum resembling a vulva (Fig. 19.21). The patient will now have to join the other half of the population and void sitting down.

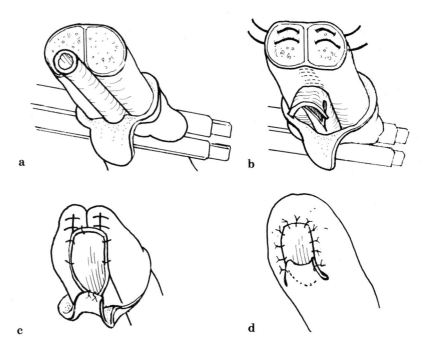

a b c d

Fig. 19.20 Localized carcinoma of the penis that recurs after radiotherapy is treated by partial amputation.

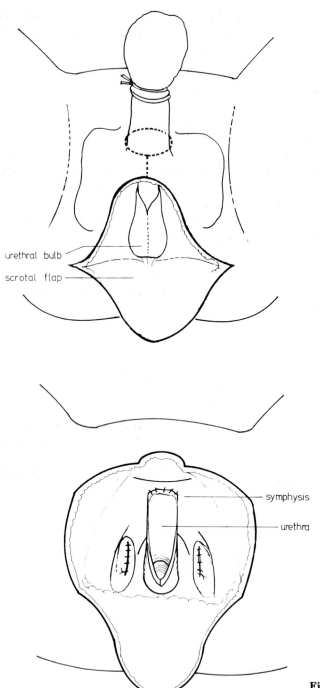

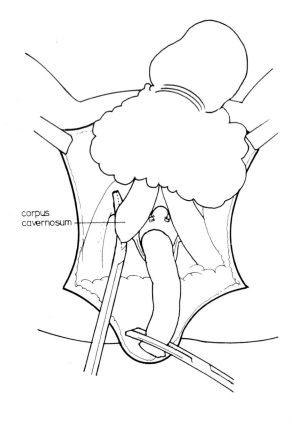

Fig. 19.21 Radical amputation for advanced carcinoma of the penis.

The preparation for operation, the postoperative care and the risks of bleeding and infection are the same as for urethroplasty (see p. 229). The catheter is removed after 3 to 4 days.

Block dissection of the inguinal nodes

When the inguinal lymph nodes are involved, block dissection is performed. This operation necessarily blocks the lymphatic pathways from the legs, which always become oedematous. The wound in the groin always leaks a considerable volume of lymph which is collected in vacuum bottles with the object of preventing secondary infection. To prevent oedema the legs are kept elevated from the first postoperative day, and the patient must wear supporting stockings for several years. We have found early use of 'Flotron' therapy to be effective.

There are times when it is necessary for the patient as well as for those who are caring for him to remind themselves that the morbidity of this swelling of the leg is the price that must be paid for cure — which can be expected in more than half of these men.

Further reading

Blandy, J. P. (1976) Penis and scrotum. In *Urology*, vol. 2, ed. Blandy, J. P., pp. 1049–1095. Blackwell Scientific Publications, Oxford.

Blandy, J. P. (1986) *Operative Urology*, 2nd edn, pp. 196-202. Blackwell Scientific Publications, Oxford.

Brindley, G. S. (1985) Pathophysiology of erection and ejaculation. In *Textbook of Genito-Urinary Surgery*, vol. 2, eds Whitfield, H. N. & Hendry, W. F., pp. 1083–1094. Churchill Livingstone, Edinburgh.

Pryor, J. P. (1985) Investigation and treatment of impotence. In *Textbook of Genito-Urinary Surgery*, vol. 2, eds Whitfield, H. N. & Hendry, W. F., pp. 1095–1108. Churchill Livingstone, Edinburgh.

20 *The testicle and scrotum*

Anatomy

The testicles lie in the scrotum — a bag supplied with a strong covering of muscle — the dartos — which is capable of contracting or relaxing to allow the testicles to hang right down or draw them up into a tight little sac. Normally the dartos is relaxed and the testicles hang down, and it is believed that this may help keep the testicles cool and promote spermatogenesis.

Each testis is an egg-shaped body, composed of rows of hollow tubules which are the production lines for the manufacture of spermatozoa. These tubules empty into the hilum of the testis from which the sperms are carried on a current of seminal plasma along vasa efferentia testis into the *epididymis* (Fig. 20.1).

The epididymis is a long coiled tube lined with cells whose hairs (*cilia*) sweep the sperms along the lumen. During this long journey most of the sperms are reabsorbed by the epididymis, which seems to act as a quality control which allows only the best ones to leave the epididymis.

Emerging from the epididymis the surviving sperms enter a long muscular pipe, the *vas deferens*, which runs up the back of the spermatic cord, winding around the inferior epigastric artery, to dive down in the

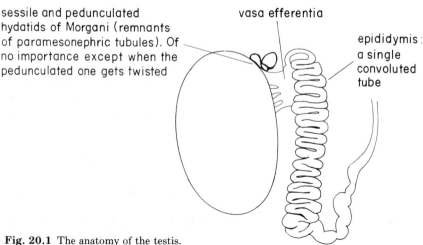

sessile and pedunculated hydatids of Morgani (remnants of paramesonephric tubules). Of no importance except when the pedunculated one gets twisted

vasa efferentia

epididymis: a single convoluted tube

Fig. 20.1 The anatomy of the testis.

1 it curls around lateral to the inferior epigastric artery in the internal inguinal ring, leaving the other contents of the spermatic cord laterally

2 it slips over the ureter at the groove between bladder and prostate

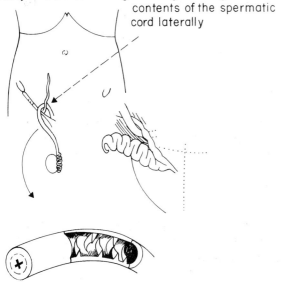

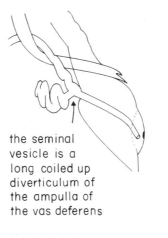

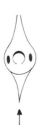

the seminal vesicle is a long coiled up diverticulum of the ampulla of the vas deferens

the verumontanum — the main landmark of the surgeon doing any operation on the prostate; middle hole is the utriculus masculinus (of no importance); each side hole is a common ejaculatory duct

note how the inside of the vas deferens is thrown up into bulkheads and folds suggesting that it is a store as well as a pulsatile duct

Fig. 20.2 The course of the vas deferens and seminal vesicle.

gap between the upper and lower zones of the prostate, to enter the urethra on the verumontanum (Fig. 20.2). Just before each vas passes between the two zones of the prostate it is joined by its *seminal vesicle* — which lies behind the upper part of the prostate.

The main function of the seminal vesicle is to supply the bulk of the seminal fluid. The first phase of ejaculation is for the vasa deferentia to empty a small bolus — about 0.5 ml — of sperms into the prostatic urethra. In the second phase the seminal vesicles squirt out another 4 or 5 ml to expel the sperms out of the urethra. The seminal vesicles manufacture fructose which sperms live on and if the seminal vesicles are diseased there is no fructose in the semen which has a very small volume.

Congenital disorders of the testicles

Undescended testicle — cryptorchidism

The testis originates in the gonadal ridge of the fetus behind the peritoneal cavity. It migrates towards the scrotum about the time of birth.

It can be held up along the course of this normal descent — *incomplete descent* — or it can wander off course and fetch up in the perineum, the thigh or at the base of the penis — *ectopic testis* (Fig. 20.3).

The descent of the testis is normally completed within a few months of birth, and if the incompletely descended testis has not reached the scrotum by the time the boy is 1 year old, it is never going to. It should therefore be operated on to bring it down as should all the ectopic ones. The operation should be done between 2 or 3 years old. Unfortunately even today diagnosis is often not made until children are much older. A testicle absent from the scrotum needs to be tracked down because of the high risk of malignancy.

Retractile testicles

In former times it was customary to wait for puberty in the belief that some of the incompletely descended testicles would come down then. This was based on a misunderstanding of the normal range of movement of the testicle (Fig. 20.4). The testicle is drawn up by the cremaster muscle which surrounds the spermatic cord under stress or in cold weather. This is a normal protective reflex, and in normal boys a fully descended testicle can often be found to be drawn right up to the external inguinal ring when he about to be examined by a strange doctor with cold fingers. These 'retractile' testicles stop riding up and down and settle in the bottom of the scrotum and they do not need an operation, but in little boys it needs

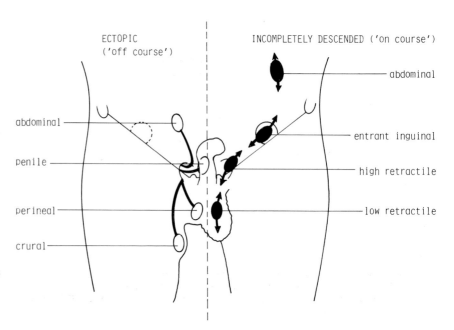

Fig. 20.3 Different types of undescended testicle; all those that are not truly 'low retractile' must be brought down surgically.

gentleness and warm hands to be sure that they are retractile rather than truly maldescended.

In former times this misunderstanding led to the use of gonadotrophic hormones in boys with maldescended testicles. Since hormones would bring on a premature puberty down would come those testicles that were going to come down anyway. The premature puberty also brought on other less desirable changes including premature closure of the vertebral epiphyses and failure to grow to full adult height.

Complications of maldescent of the testicle

TORSION OF THE TESTIS

The undescended testis often has a very baggy peritoneal sac in front of it, the *processus vaginalis* in which the testicle may twist on a pedicle (Fig. 20.5) so tightly that it cuts off its blood supply; this is *torsion of the testis*. It can occur at any age, most often around puberty. Although is particularly likely to occur in undescended testes, it is also seen in those that are fully descended.

Typically the patient give a story of previous episodes of pain in the testicle — suddenly coming on — suddenly going away. Sometimes a boy will wake with the pain and within an hour or so the testicle has become red and swollen. If seen early, it can sometimes be untwisted manually

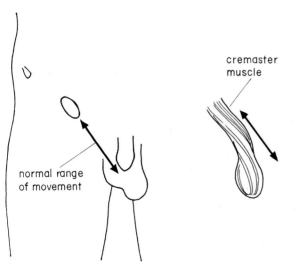

Fig. 20.4 The normal testicle may be drawn up towards the external inguinal ring by the cremaster muscle; this normal range of movement must be distinguished from true maldescent.

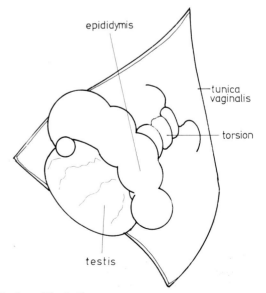

Fig. 20.5 Torsion of the testis.

after a full dose of pethidine. Usually it must be explored as an emergency: if untwisted in time, the testicle may be saved. The underlying extra baggy tunica vaginalis which allows torsion to occur is often present on the other side, so both testes are always explored to prevent similar torsion of the other testicle.

INFERTILITY

Maldescent of both testicles is accompanied by a very much decreased chance of fertility, but unilateral maldescent is of no consequence.

CANCER

Cancer of the testicle is more common in men with a history of cryptorchidism. It may affect the other, normally descended testis. If cancer arises in a testicle that has remained inside the abdomen, it has often spread before the malignancy is detected, and every male with a testicle that is not found in the inguinal canal is advised to undergo laparotomy to seek and remove the undescended gonad and quite often carcinoma *in situ* is found in these testicles.

Orchidopexy

The operation to bring down the testicle is performed through a short incision over the internal inguinal ring (Fig. 20.6). The inguinal canal is

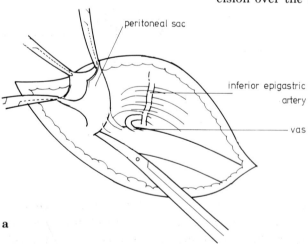

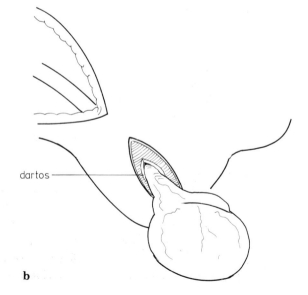

Fig. 20.6 Orchidopexy: when the spermatic cord is detached from the back of the peritoneum the testicle is brought down into a pouch between the skin and the dartos muscle of the scrotum.

opened; the processus vaginalis is separated from the spermatic cord, freeing the cord from the back of the peritoneum, until the testicle can be placed in a pocket between the dartos and the scrotal skin. There will be small incisions in the groin and scrotum.

Hydrocele

The normal space of the processus vaginalis around the testicle contains a trace of fluid which allows the testis to move around within the scrotum, obviously a useful protection against minor injury. If the lymphatics draining the testicle are obstructed, this fluid increases, to produce a bag — a *hydrocele* that surrounds the front and sides of the testicle. A similar effusion of fluid occurs if the testicle is diseased, for example with cancer. Most hydroceles are idiopathic — i.e. nobody knows why.

Tapping a hydrocele

The fluid may be aspirated repeatedly, using a plastic cannula as used for intravenous infusions (Fig. 20.7); a minor procedure which can be performed in the outpatient clinic. If the fluid fills up again quickly, an operation to cure the hydrocele is performed (Fig. 20.8). The processus vaginalis is removed and its edge sewn up to stop bleeding.

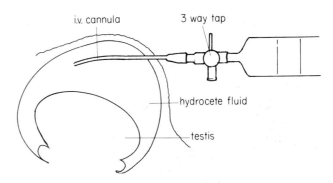

Fig. 20.7 Tapping a hydrocele.

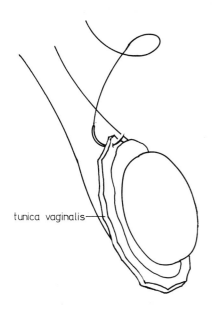

Fig. 20.8 Radical cure of a hydrocele.

A preoperative shave is necessary. Afterwards a firm scrotal support or firm underpants are worn. Nearly always the scrotum becomes very swollen for a few weeks after operations for hydrocele — often much larger than it was before and the patient may become quite anxious, fearing that something has gone wrong. Explain that this is quite normal and that it will take a few weeks for the swelling to subside.

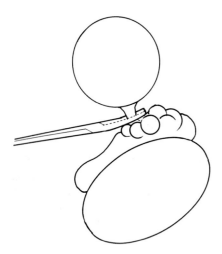

Fig. 20.9 Removing a cyst of the epididymis.

Cysts of the epididymis

There are often little out-pouchings of the vasa efferentia testis — the tubes that convey the sperms from the rete testis to the epididymis. They may continue to enlarge until they form a collection of little cysts containing seminal plasma. This is usually a clear watery fluid but may contain sperms — sometimes so many as to make the fluid look like cream — hence the old name *spermatocele*. Small cysts of the epididymis are almost always present in men after the age of 30 and only need treatment if they become so large that the patient is uncomfortable. They can be aspirated but this is seldom successful or comfortable for the patient, and as a rule they are excised — a procedure which is similar to that for the radical cure of a hydrocele (Fig. 20.9).

Injury of the testis

The testis can be ruptured by an injury in sport or at work. There is a split in the visceral layer of the tunica vaginalis (Fig. 20.10). Blood leaks and fills up the sac to form a *haematocele*. If neglected, this blood clot organizes, swells and compresses the testicle and eventually leads to atrophy. Injured testicles must be explored as an emergency; the blood is evacuated and the torn tunica sewn up. By doing this the function of the testis can be saved. This type of injury is very painful: rest and analgesics are needed, as well as support for the scrotum.

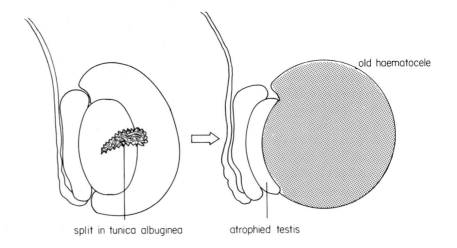

split in tunica albuginea   atrophied testis

Fig. 20.10 In injury of the testis unless the haematoma is removed it may compress the testis and lead to atrophy.

Acute orchitis

Mumps

Mumps occurs in epidemics and the well known parotitis is its usual manifestation. In adults the testicles may be affected — a disease which can be very painful. It does not occur in boys before puberty, and even during a mumps epidemic torsion of the testicle is a much more probable diagnosis when a schoolboy has an acutely swollen testis. When in doubt these cases should be explored. Decompression of the testicle by incising the tunica vaginalis may prevent the atrophy that all too often follows mumps orchitis.

Bacterial infection — epididymo-orchitis

1 Secondary to urinary infection, it presents with a painful swelling at first limited to the epididymis, but later making the whole testicle swell.
2 In many men however no urinary organisms can be found, and tuberculosis must always be suspected, and ruled out by culturing three early morning specimens of urine (see p. 52).

Whatever its cause, in epididymitis the patient has severe pain and needs analgesics and rest. A scrotal support may be worn after the first few days. Antibiotic treatment must be continued for up to 6 weeks. Many patients give a history of having been doing some unusually heavy lifting just before the onset of the pain and swelling in the epididymis, suggesting that urine may have been forced back along the vas deferens to the epididymis. In any event, heavy lifting must be forbidden until the epididymitis has resolved.

In some men repeated attacks of epididymitis can be so disabling and so frequent that it is necessary to perform vasectomy to divide the link between the urinary tract and the epididymis, or even remove the entire epididymis.

Occasionally epididymitis will suppurate and an abscess forms. This is very serious: it needs to be incised, and sometimes part of the necrotic testicle may be extruded along with the contents of the abscess as a 'fungus testis' and when this occurs the testicle has to be removed.

In *tuberculous epididymitis* the disease may also be present in the prostate, seminal vesicles, kidneys and bladder. The treatment is along the usual lines for tuberculosis (see p. 53). Sometimes it is necessary to remove the epididymis.

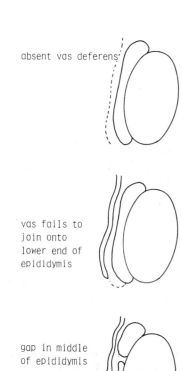

absent vas deferens

vas fails to
join onto
lower end of
epididymis

gap in middle
of epididymis

Fig. 20.11 Infertility may result from the congenital failure of union of vas and epididymis.

Male infertility

Congenital causes

Both testes may be absent or maldescended; such patients have no sperms in the semen at all and biopsy of the undescended testes show that there are no germinal cells in the tubules from which the sperms originate. In addition, there is often a failure of union between the vas deferens and the epididymis (Fig. 20.11).

Trauma

The vas deferens may be divided by accident at an operation for a hernia or an undescended testicle. If so it can be joined up again with a good chance of success.

Inflammation

Mumps may destroy the testicle but is usually limited to one testis. Gonorrhoea causes a stenosis where the vas deferens joins the epididymis. It can be overcome by *epididymovasostomy*.

Through a scrotal incision the vas is freed up and sewn side to side to the epididymis upstream of the blockage (Fig. 20.12).

Varicocele

The veins draining the testicle are often very large in otherwise healthy young men. There is a widespread belief that patients with a supposedly 'low' sperm count will be made better if the varicocele is operated on, and although every carefully controlled study has refuted this idea, the operation is still widely practised.

Through a short incision just above the inguinal canal the testicular veins are found just lateral to the inferior epigastric artery (Fig. 20.13). The veins are separated from the artery and divided between ligatures.

Vasectomy

The patient and his partner must clearly understand that once divided, it is very difficult to put the vasa together again successfully; they must continue to use other contraceptive measures until all the sperms have disappeared from the semen; and that there is a remote chance that the divided vasa may spontaneously join together again months or years later. Specially worded forms for 'consent for operation' are completed.

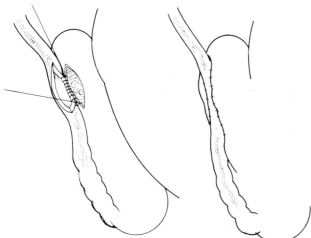

Fig. 20.12 Epididymovasostomy.

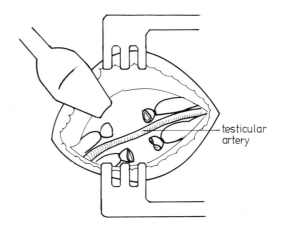

testicular
artery

Fig. 20.13 Operation for varicocele: the testicular veins are separated from the artery just above the inguinal ligament, ligated, and divided.

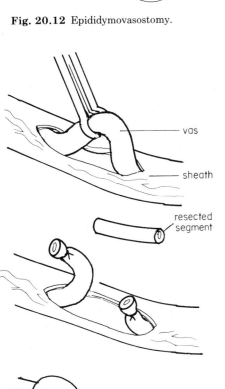

vas

sheath

resected
segment

Fig. 20.14 Vasectomy.

Vasectomy is often performed under local anaesthetic as an out-patient. Before he comes up, the patient should have shaved the area and had a bath.

It is important to appreciate that this, like any other 'minor' operation, must not be done unless certain precautions are at hand. Traction on the vas causes stimulation of the vagus nerve in a number of patients. As a result the heart may slow down, and even stop. Hence wherever vasectomy is being performed there must be the minimum equipment available for resuscitation (see p. 24).

After infiltrating with local anaesthetic, a short incision is made over the vas deferens. The vas is lifted up, infiltrated with more local anaesthetic, and then divided (Fig. 20.14). Many procedures are used in the hope of preventing spontaneous reunion of the vasa. Some surgeons turn one end back on itself; some try to bury the cut ends in tissue; others coagulate the ends of the vasa with diathermy to seal them off. After careful haemostasis the little incision is closed.

Reactionary haemorrhage must be anticipated: small veins in the scrotal skin which were closed as a result of spasm during the dissection may relax afterwards allowing blood to collect in the soft tissues of the scrotum — a haematoma. For this reason patients should be allowed to rest quietly for 10 to 15 minutes after the operation, and the scrotum should be inspected before they go home. Reactionary haemorrhage may occur up to 2 or 3 hours later and it is always necessary that the patient knows who to telephone for help.

It can take many months before the sperms have all disappeared from the storage system of the vas deferens, the ampulla and the seminal vesicles. As nobody can tell how long sperms may remain alive and capable of fertilizing an ovum it is the rule to examine the semen repeatedly until two consecutive specimens of semen have shown no sperms at all in a centrifuged specimen. In the meantime contraceptive precautions must be continued. Recently cases have been reported where, months or years after the vasectomy the vasa have joined together again spontaneously, a phenomenon which was believed to be impossible. Nowadays patients are warned of this possibility which is about as likely as winning the football pools; nevertheless they need to know that it might occur.

Rejoining the vas after vasectomy

More and more men return several years after the vasectomy asking to have their vasa put together again, sometimes because of the tragic death of children, sometimes because they have remarried. It is not difficult to do (Fig. 20.15) but it requires a more extended dissection than the original vasectomy, and so a general anaesthetic is needed. Many surgeons use the operating microscope to help rejoin these tiny tubes.

A preoperative shave is performed. After the operation the patient needs a firm scrotal support which should be worn for a week. He can go home 2 or 3 days after the operation, but he should then rest and should not return to work for 2 weeks. The semen may be examined for the return of sperms from about 3 months after the operation but it may take up to 2 years before the operation can be seen to have been successful.

The results are disappointing. Although about 80% of reanastomoses are followed by appearance of sperms in the ejaculate, unfortunately only about 50% of these men father children. The reason is not clear: it may be that antibodies are formed against sperms as a result of the prolonged blockage and the increased activity of the epididymes.

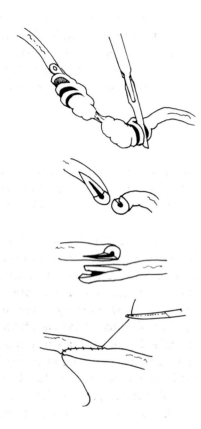

Fig. 20.15 Re-anastomosis of the vas deferens.

Cancer of the testis

This is one of the real success stories in the treatment of cancer. Instead of being a certain death sentence, testicular cancer today can nearly always be cured no matter how advanced the disease when first detected. Knowing this can be of enormous help in providing the encouragement that is often so badly needed in the months of therapy that may be necessary.

Cancer presents as a lump in the testis (Fig. 20.16). An ultrasound scan may be used if there is any doubt about the diagnosis. After blood has

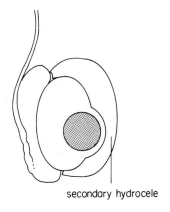

secondary hydrocele

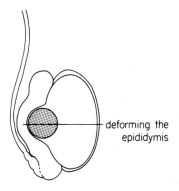

deforming the
epididymis

Fig. 20.16 Any solid lump in the body of the testis must be suspected of being a cancer.

been taken for the measurement of *tumour markers*, minute amounts of alpha-feto protein and beta-human chorionic gonadotrophin that are secreted by some of the cancer cells, the patient should have the testicle explored. If it is found to be malignant, the spermatic cord is ligated and divided at the internal inguinal ring by the operation of *inguinal orchidectomy* (Fig. 20.17).

Staging for testicular cancer

Testicular cancers spread to the lymph nodes high up the aorta at the level of the renal arteries (Fig. 20.18). A careful search is made for enlargement of these lymph nodes by means of a CT scan (Fig. 20.19) or a lymphangiogram (Fig. 20.20).

The *lymphangiogram* is an unpleasant investigation for the patient. The dorsum of each foot is shaved. A few ml of a green dye which stings a little is injected between the toes, and is taken up into the lymphatics. They are exposed through a short incision made under local anaesthesia in the dorsum of each foot and a small cannula inserted through which an oily contrast medium is slowly injected. The oil runs up the lymphatics and fills the lymph nodes. If they are invaded by cancer there is a filling defect. Warn your patient that this is a very tedious investigation which takes hours and he should take a good book with him to the X-ray department. Warn him also that his skin will take on a greenish-blue tinge and his urine will be stained green for a day or two afterwards. Further X-rays with an IVU are taken 48 hours afterwards.

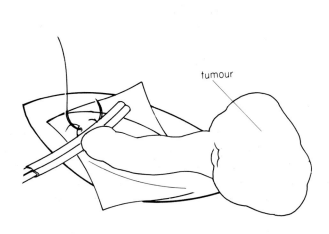

tumour

Fig. 20.17 Inguinal orchidectomy.

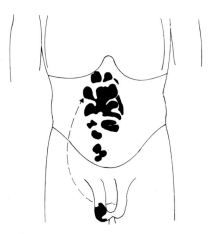

Fig. 20.18 Testicular cancer spreads to the para-aortic lymph nodes. Note that inguinal lymph nodes are not involved unless previous surgery has been done in the groin, e.g. hernia or orchidectomy.

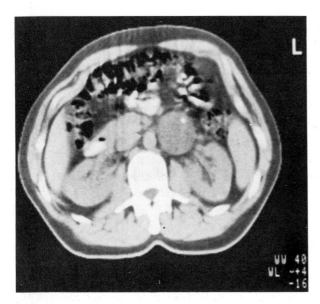

Fig. 20.19 CT scan showing enlarged lymph nodes in the para-aortic region.

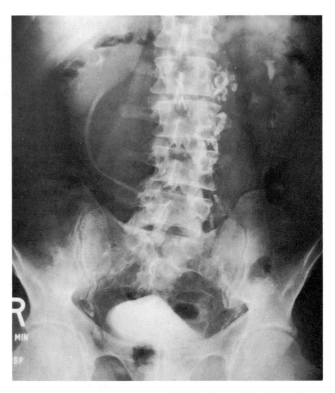

Fig. 20.20 Lymphangiogram and IVP: a large mass of tumour in the right para-aortic nodes has displaced the ureter and prevented contrast medium from entering the lymph nodes.

Nowadays the battery of screening tests available for testicular cancer is very accurate. If no cancer can be found in the CT scan or lymphangiogram, and if the markers are negative, selected patients are kept under *surveillance*, i.e. they are very carefully watched, and the investigations are repeated at intervals to make sure that no tumour appears.

If the tests reveal cancer in the retroperitoneal nodes, the patient is given a course of *chemotherapy* using various combinations of cis-platinum, bleomycin, vinblastine and other agents. The treatment is unpleasant and must only be given under strict supervision by a well-trained team. The side-effects include bone marrow suppression, loss of hair, and dreadful vomiting — though this can be controlled by drugs, much understanding and support are needed. But the cancer disappears, and the patients are cured.

When the tests show large masses of widespread tumour, the first line of treatment is chemotherapy, but sometimes the lumps do not entirely

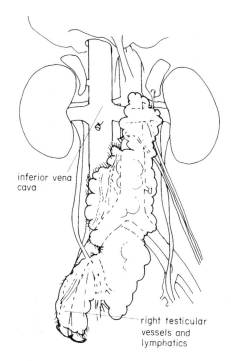

inferior vena
cava

right testicular
vessels and
lymphatics

Fig. 20.21 Radical retroperitoneal lymph node dissection.

disappear and the patient is left with a mass in the abdomen and an unsolved question: is it all dead fibrous tissue or is living cancer still present? One cannot afford to take chances, and these patients are now explored, and the mass removed.

The operation is prolonged and difficult (Fig. 20.21). Through a long midline incision the bowel is completely mobilized and packed away out of the abdomen. All the tissue surrounding the aorta and inferior vena cava is dissected clear leaving only the great vessels, kidneys and ureters behind. Following the operation these patients have 2 or 3 days of ileus, but generally recover surprisingly quickly. If the lump is found to contain only necrotic fibrous tissue, the patients can be considered to be cured. If one finds only 'benign teratoma' tissue — i.e. the chemotherapy has converted the cancer into a benign precursor, then the outlook is also excellent so long as all the mass has been removed, for within a few years this 'benign teratoma' will otherwise revert to a malignant state. If any active cancer is found in the tissue the patient will need further chemotherapy. This is a very extensive operation and it can be very encouraging for the patient to know that it is very much worthwhile. In *seminoma* the cancer is so sensitive to chemotherapy that smaller and less toxic doses may be given. It is also very sensitive to radiotherapy, and rather than run the slight risk of recurrence most units prefer to give these patients a low dose of irradiation as a prophylactic measure.

Further reading

Atwell, J. D. & Ellis, H. (1961) Rupture of the testis. *British Journal of Surgery*, **49**, 345–346.

Bates, T. D. (1985) Management of testicular tumours. *Journal of the Royal Society of Medicine*, **78** (Suppl. 6), 1–47.

Blackmore, C. A. (1985) *The Impact of Orchidectomy Upon the Male With Testicular Cancer*. Royal Marsden Publication 586. DHSS, London.

Blandy, J. P. (1976) Testicular neoplasms. In *Urology*, vol. 2, ed Blandy, J. P., pp. 1203–1230. Blackwell Scientific Publications, Oxford.

Blandy, J. P. (1986) *Operative Urology*, 2nd edn, pp. 238–254. Blackwell Scientific Publications, Oxford.

Lange, P. (ed.) (1984) Testicular carcinoma. *World Journal of Urology*, **2**, 1–86.

Oliver, R. T. D., Hope-Stone, H. F. & Blandy, J. P. (1984) Possible new approaches to the management of seminoma of the testis. *British Journal of Urology*, **56**, 729–733.

Oliver, R. T. D., Blandy, J. P. & Hope-Stone, H. F. (1984) Controversies concerning the management of germ-cell tumors. In *World Urology Update Series*, vol. 2, lesson 1, pp. 1–7. Continuing Professional Education Center (CPEC), New Jersey.

Whitaker, R. H. (1976) Benign disorders of the testicle. In *Urology*, vol. 2, ed. Blandy, J. P., pp. 1179–1202. Blackwell Scientific Publications, Oxford.

Index